Dirk Schweigler

IBS and digestive disorders

from a totally new perspective

The author has carefully selected and reviewed the advice provided in this book. However, it should in no way replace getting competent medical advice. All information in this book is therefore provided without any warranty or guarantee of any kind on the part of the author. The author's liability for personal injury, property damage and financial loss is also excluded.

First edition 2023

Illustrations: *Shutterstock*
Translation: *Mary Burdman, PA, USA*

Table of contents

Introduction

The name "IBS" will definitely not make it into the Top 10 list of great disease-names. However, you don't pick your diseases voluntarily like you select your shoes or the next destination for your vacation. On the other hand, diseases don't simply come out of the blue; they don´t come unexpectedly and for no reason. There is always a cause behind it, even if we cannot always recognize this cause at first glance.

The acronym IBS stands for **I**rritable **B**owel **S**yndrome and you can notice it from the typical symptoms like stomach cramps, bloating, diarrhea or constipation. But even when you get the diagnosis "irritable bowel syndrome," that won´t help you much. This diagnosis only means that your bowel is irritated and most people already know by themselves that their bowel is not working well, because they feel it every day. What really matters for anyone who has digestive problems, is the question of why their bowel is irritated and what you can do about it.

I have announced in the title that this book will show a totally new perspective on IBS as well as on digestive problems in general and you are probably asking yourself what this completely new vantage point is supposed to mean. I have been struggling with digestive problems for a long time and since doctors couldn´t help me with my problems, I had to do all the homework myself: I read a lot of books on the issue and did intensive research.

After a while, I noticed that the vast majority of books or websites about this topic only deal with how to avoid certain foods or how you can live with your digestion problems. But the end result is always the same: You have to put up with these digestive disorders for the rest of your life.

I would therefore like to take a look at the IBS issue from a completely new vantage point – from the perspective of the **causes**. This means, you should not be concerned about how you come to terms with digestive problems for the rest of your life. Instead, the aim is to make it possible to rid yourself of food intolerances. It´s a very simple idea and it works for almost all diseases: When you heal the cause of a disease, then the symptoms disappear all on their own. But it simply doesn't work the other way around – working on the symptoms won´t heal the cause.

The idea for the title "IBS and digestive disorders from a totally new perspective" came from the movie "Vantage Point." In this movie, the heads of state of several countries meet for an anti-terrorist summit. At this meeting, there is an assassination attempt against the U.S. president and the movie continues telling the story from eight different perspectives: From the perspective of a woman reporter, a police officer, a spectator, from the perspective of the U.S. president and from the perspective of the instigators of the terrorist act.

I find this approach very interesting because a story isn't the only thing that we can see from several vantage points, but a disease also has several perspectives. And therefore, I would like to bring the focus to the causes of IBS. The causes are considered far too rarely, even though they are the root of the problem.

If you go a little deeper into the subject of irritable bowel syndrome, then you suddenly find yourself stumbling upon terms such as "alpha-1 antitrypsin" or "pancreatic elastase" and you end up dealing with tongue-twisters in addition to your damaged intestine. Even so, it is important that you have heard these terms and laboratory names at least once. You won't be able to show off with this knowledge at the next dinner party because most healthy people simply aren't very interested in this. The main reason why it is so important to understand these medical terms is that you can always take care of your recovery yourself and support your body, with whatever it needs. But in order to do this, you need sufficient specialist knowledge. Most persons affected by digestive problems have had the experience that their doctors simply cannot help much when it comes to healing these problems.

There are two main reasons for that: For most doctors, their time per patient is very much limited. And the second reason is that the majority of doctors are focusing on dealing with the symptoms instead of looking at the root cause. One possible cause of IBS can be an imbalance of your gut bacteria, and this recalls the situation of a few years ago, when most doctors fiercely denied that anything such as gut bacteria even existed at all.

At that time, most of the developments concerning the good gut bacteria came from alternative practitioners, and at that time gut bacteria were mostly labeled hocus-pocus. Scientific laboratories have offered tests for many years now to check the status of the intestine, such as inflammation as well as the bacterial status.

I remember the times when antibiotics where prescribed in bulk by doctors paying very little attention to the side effects. Fortunately, this has changed now and meanwhile, gut bacteria have even become the subject of intensive research in conventional medicine. Therefore, I am assuming and hoping that the topic of IBS will also get more attention from conventional medicine in due course.

I myself have a very long medical odyssey behind me. In fact, that's something many patients experience, as you run from one doctor to another and nobody can really help you out. My first digestive problems set in while I was still completing my studies. But that was all within the scope of what was tolerable, especially since digestive problems tend to sneak up on you, slowly and gradually. It is only in the very rarest cases that you wake up one day with food intolerances and an irritable bowel, although you were totally healthy the evening before. In most cases, you will develop more and more intolerances slowly over time, especially if you don't do anything about them.

After completing my studies, I lived in India for more than a year in order to master the Hindu scriptures. It was an incredibly exciting time because India is so totally different in almost every way. However, the bacteria and the hygiene standards are also totally different and I caught really serious gastrointestinal infections several times. There were situations when the temperature outside was very hot, but I was lying in bed with chills and covered with a thick blanket and I knew that things just hadn't been fine with the meal I ate the day before.

Within a few days, I recovered from these gastrointestinal infections, but in their wake came a free membership in the irritable bowel club. At that point in time, I didn't know what to do about it. After I returned home back to Germany, I was only able to eat about six to eight foods, such as rice, potatoes, oatmeal, bread rolls and broccoli. At this point I realized that I urgently had to do something about this situation.

The first port of call was my general practitioner, but he only recommended fennel-anise-caraway tea. That was all he knew about it. Therefore, the next step was to go directly to a gastrointestinal specialist. Here, I thought, I am really at the right place and he can certainly fix my irritable bowel. The mandatory colonoscopy was performed. Everything was great – I was officially healthy and could go home. Supposedly, I should actually have been glad that there was nothing worse behind the symptoms. Nevertheless, I was anything but satisfied, because nothing had changed at all in terms of my symptoms.

After I had consulted four doctors, I slowly realized that conventional medicine couldn´t help me much here. Then the next stop was the "Institute for Food Intolerances" in Hamburg. The concept there is that you spit into a container for two hours and afterwards you are prescribed something based on that data. Allegedly, a reprogramming of the immune system had taken place. To make it short: This is pure hocus-pocus and simply doesn't work. Well, it actually does work, but only for the doctors there who earn quite a lot of money in this process. For the patients, such useless treatment does nothing to make you better in any way – only your wallet definitely becomes lighter.

This method just can´t work, because over 90% of people with irritable bowel syndrome have no problems at all with their immune system. Instead, the problems can be traced back to gut bacteria, candida fungi, heavy metal toxicity, infections or histamine intolerance. But it is only in the rarest of cases that this has anything to do with the immune system. When the immune system reacts to certain foods, that would be an allergy and these are significantly much rarer in comparison to food intolerances.

For me, further visits to a naturopathic practitioner and a TCM practitioner were unsuccessful. They definitely took considerably more time with me and gave my digestive system support in a natural way, which is a good thing at first. But this also didn't bring any real improvement. Until I came across a naturopathic practitioner who understood his craft properly. As a result, we looked more closely at the location where the problem lay – the intestine. Only the method of approach was different. In a colonoscopy, the intestine is also observed, but more at its surface. However, the key thing is to go to a more specific micro-level. And that can be done wonderfully by taking a **stool sample** which is then examined by a certified laboratory.

With this stool sample, I had a very concrete result for the first time. It was no longer a matter of diffuse problems along the lines of "*There is something or other I can't tolerate*" but rather, I finally had a specific diagnosis. Once you have a diagnosis, then you can follow it up by starting a very concrete treatment.

If my long quest to find a solution for my digestive problems were something extremely rare, then I would have kept it to myself, happily enjoying that things are fine now. But during my long journey, while I visited doctors or researched on the Internet, I met so many people out there with a very similar story. They had also been looking for years to find someone who could help them with their digestive problems.

In the meantime, I can now eat almost all foods again and have hardly any restrictions. Unfortunately, during my long search for a solution, I also tried a lot of things that were completely useless. Now in retrospect, I understand why nothing really worked for me. The majority of doctors I have visited only focused on my symptoms and they have never really searched for the root cause. Left alone with my problems, I started taking randomly “something” against my digestive disorders and this didn´t help me either, because I disregarded a very important principle.

Before buying any product for "digestive problems," you need to do a precise diagnosis first. You always need to stick to the basic principle: **First the diagnosis, then the therapy!**

To spare you having to take the long road through many failed attempts and the associated costs, I would like to make all of my knowledge available in this book. Having knowledge about the right treatment is similar to taking a vacation trip: When you have a map, you can get straight to your destination. Without a map, on the other hand, you wander around aimlessly and you have to try taking many different directions before you get to your destination – if you ever arrive. For treating IBS, this aimless wandering not only costs you time, it can also cost a lot of money, many years of pain and an enormously restricted life – every day. Unfortunately, I know all of this too well from my own experience.

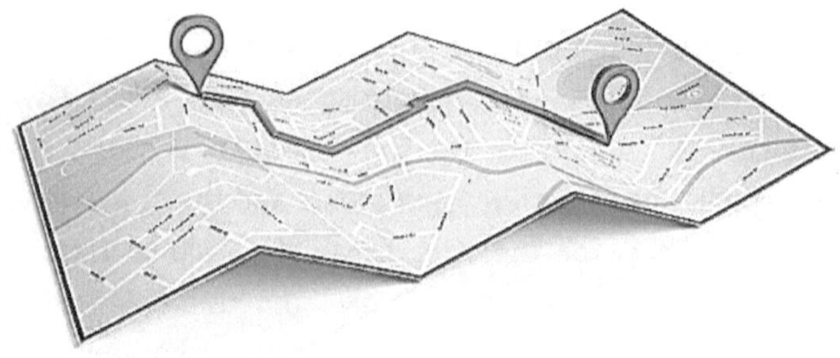

All the measures and tests that I will introduce here are ones I have tested and used myself. It isn't possible to state generally for everyone who has digestive disorders what the cause is. This is because there are simply too many different causes that come into question. But I will try to provide you with enough knowledge so that you can easily determine the cause of your IBS. It isn´t even that difficult, because nowadays there are a vast number of great scientific tests which make it possible to find out what is causing the digestive problems.

When treating digestive problems, just taking a whack at the symptoms with a mallet doesn't help at all. That means, for example, prescribing medications for diarrhea that only slow down the action of the bowel. Another example is administering remedies for flatulence (gas) which only dissolve the air bubbles in the intestine.

Such measures cannot be called treatment. Instead, they merely represent the suppression of symptoms. And as soon as the medication is discontinued, the problems come back. In the following, we don't want to deal just with the symptoms, but above all we will deal with the causes. If you can cure the cause, the symptoms disappear on their own and never come back.

You can compare the cause and symptoms of a disease with a warning light in a car. If your car has too little oil in its engine, the oil warning light comes on brightly on the display. But the warning light is only the symptom. The underlying cause is the lack of oil. In order to get your car driving well, you have to take care of the lack of oil instead of working on the warning lamp.

You can also ignore the warning light. Then the underlying cause (the lack of oil) persists or even gets worse. And when dealing with a car, nobody would come up with the idea of tinkering with the symptoms, such as by taping over the warning light. You go to the engine and fix the cause by just filling it up with oil and then the oil warning light goes out all by itself.

And this is exactly how you should deal with IBS: You don't concentrate on the symptoms – that is, not on the warning light. Rather, it is the underlying causes that are decisive and therefore we will take a closer look at all the possible causes that should be taken under consideration.

Since I have worked as a scientist at a university hospital for several years, I attach great importance to taking a scientific approach, particularly to medical issues. At the same time, I also believe that we should not simply throw many centuries of experience overboard.

For example, if the herbs lavender or valerian have already helped our great-grandparents to fall asleep easily, then you can rely on this experience with a clear conscience. And if there is a medical study that proves this scientifically, so much the better. Therefore, scientific method and experience should go hand in hand. Unfortunately, ancient knowledge sometimes is just forgotten or ignored nowadays.

Another important aspect of the therapy is that there is no standard way that works for everybody. Every person has a totally individual body and each person has experienced completely different events in the past that led to their digestive problems. Unfortunately, I have to disappoint all those who were hoping that there would be this one amazing pill. This doesn´t exist, simply because there are way too many different causes for it to be considered.

Investigating multiple causes may sound complicated at first, but in fact this is not the case at all. Step by step, we will take a look at all the potential triggers for IBS. I will show you how you can test for each trigger and, of course, how this problem can be cured.

1 The starting point: A closer look into your intestine

For anyone who wants to find the cause of their digestive problems, the diagnosis is the first and most important step. Only then can an appropriate treatment follow. The symptoms, like diarrhea, flatulence, constipation or abdominal pain, will not give a definite indication about the root cause. Therefore, it takes a little more than just looking at the symptoms.

The best way to start is by examining a **stool sample**. You can get a test kit from a doctor or natural practitioner. The stool sample is then simply sent to a laboratory, where many different values can be measured. Unfortunately, most scientific laboratory terms are quite unwieldy and have almost nothing in common with the words we use every day. Often only doctors or laboratory staff are familiar with such terms. However, these lab values pack a punch, because they show exactly what is going on in the intestine and they indicate which treatment is necessary.

Any presumption, such as "I could possibly have this or that" without a diagnosis from the laboratory does not help things along. Without clear laboratory results, matters are reduced to purely speculating about which disease is behind the digestive disorders.

In order to get a complete overview of what is going on in your intestine, you should check multiple stool values at a time. From just one stool sample, it is possible to learn a great deal about how well your intestine is doing.

A complete stool analysis should therefore include the following laboratory values:

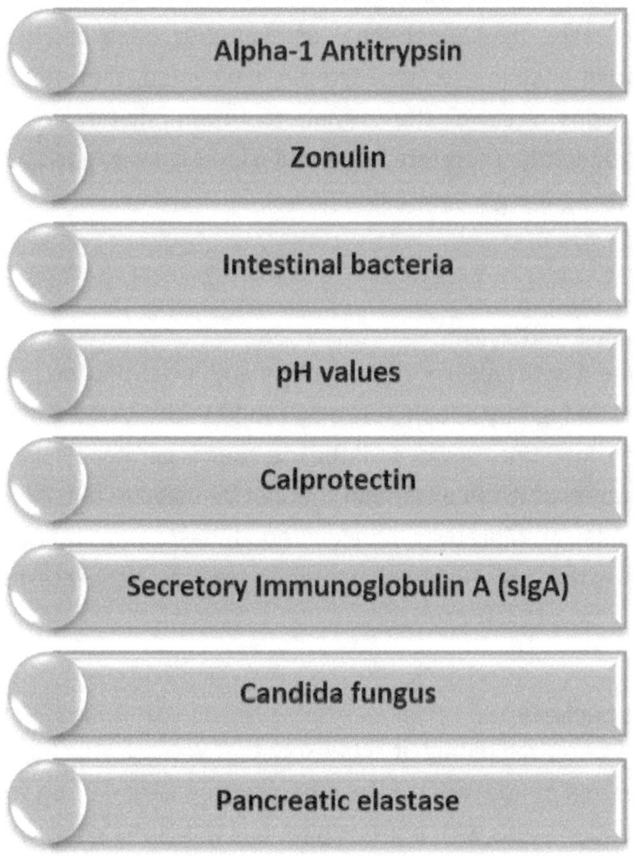

A conclusive overall picture of the condition of the intestine only emerges when all these values are taken together. It is therefore advisable to have all these laboratory values checked together from one stool sample and not to omit any values in the process. Let´s take a closer look at them:

Zonulin

Zonulin is a protein and gives a signal to the cell junctions – also called tight junctions – so that they open up. If the zonulin level in the stool sample is elevated, then the cell junctions receive the signal to open themselves up permanently. Therefore, the zonulin level is a very good basis for recognizing a permeable bowel.

Alpha-1 antitrypsin

Alpha-1 antitrypsin is also a protein and it is produced in the liver. In healthy people it is only found in the blood and not in the intestine. However, if the intestine is permeable, larger amounts of it can enter and this can be measured in a stool sample [2]. Moreover, an elevated alpha-1 antitrypsin level shows that there is an inflammation present in the intestine.

Gut bacteria

While you are eating, it is unlikely that you ask yourself the question of how will this food be digested later. For us, food ingestion stops with our last bite, but this is the point when the actual digestive work is just beginning. When it comes to digestion, we can count on the aid of many billions of little helpers. We could not exist without gut bacteria and it would be impossible to digest the food we have eaten.

In addition to their main job of digestion, gut bacteria also perform many other important tasks. About 80 percent of the entire human immune system is found in the intestine. Since the immune system is involved in many processes in the body, gut bacteria thus play a very important role from an immunological point of view.

Moreover, gut bacteria are responsible for the formation of vitamins, especially the B vitamins such as B1, B2 and B12. They have an influence on how your weight develops and they play a central role above all in patients with inflammatory intestinal diseases such as Crohn's disease or ulcerative colitis.

The *"lactobacilli"* and the *"bifidobacteria"* are the numerically largest and best-known species. Nevertheless, there are many more species present in the intestine than just these two. It is therefore important when you are taking any supplement containing gut bacteria, that it contains many different strains of bacteria which represent a wide spectrum. By ingesting gut bacteria, you are not only establishing good bacteria species in the intestine, but at the same time the bad bacteria are suppressed.

pH value

The pH value is an important prerequisite for the smooth functioning of many processes in the intestine. When the pH level is less than 7, we speak of an “acidic” state, exactly 7 is called “neutral” and greater than 7 is a “basic” state of the intestine.

When we speak generally about someone being over-acidified, this usually refers to the pH value in the urine. That is the case when the pH level in the urine is on average below 7.0. However, each organ in the body has an individual pH value. In the stomach, an extremely low pH of around 1.0 to 1.5 prevails. The intestine has a different optimal value which ranges from 5.8 to 6.5. The pH value in the intestine is very important because many good gut bacteria only feel well in this environment. In contrast, the bad bacteria multiply well at an alkaline value of more than 7.0. It is very important to keep the intestinal pH level within a good range over the long term, since you want your good bacteria to feel happy and settle down in your intestine.

Calprotectin

Calprotectin levels can be used to determine the presence of a chronic inflammatory bowel disease such as Crohn's disease or ulcerative colitis. Calprotectin is a protein that binds calcium and zinc. In addition to inflammatory bowel diseases, elevated calprotectin levels can also be due to infections or tumor diseases. In case of an elevated calprotectin level, a colonoscopy by a gastroenterologist is recommended and can provide further information.

Secretory immunoglobulin A (sIgA)

The body has built up a highly complex immune system to defend itself from unwanted external influences. It is a kind of defensive wall against intruders such as bad bacteria, viruses or parasites. Since the immune system is not a visible organ, for the most part you cannot envisage much about it.

More than 80 percent of this defense system is located in the intestine alone, thus making it the immune system's headquarters. Therefore, the intestine's condition, in terms of its health, has a very large impact on the performance of the immune system. But it can also work the other way around: A weakened immune system can have a negative effect on the intestine.

Due to the fact that the predominant part of the immune system is located in the intestine, any viral disease, for example, will affect the immune system and can therefore lead to digestive problems. Secretory immunoglobulin (SIgA) represents a good parameter for checking the activity of the immune system in the intestine. The immune system already starts working on its own, using these phenomena with tongue-twisting names.

SIgA values can move in both directions beyond the reference range and can thus be either too high or too low. A too-high SIgA value can indicate an inflammation of the intestinal mucosa or that the immune system is very active and it has to deal with viruses or parasites.

In contrast, a low SIgA value may indicate an increased susceptibility to infections or it can point to an allergic reaction like food allergies, asthma or neurodermatitis.

As a teenager, I used to catch colds very often. When I started my military service, I was very afraid that I would be sick all the time, because it was winter back then and we only had thin jackets and weren´t allowed to wear a scarf. To my surprise, I never caught a single cold and my immune system was extremely strong during that time. The key, that my immune system improved so much was, that I have been outside in the fresh air all the time. So, when you want to improve a low SIgA value and get your immune system running well again, then fresh air can really do a lot here.

Candida

Candida is a yeast that spreads mainly on the mucous membranes. The most common species is the candida albicans. In principle, it is often argued that it isn't necessary to measure candida concentrations in patients with digestive problems, because it is present in almost every person anyway. However, dealing with candida is not a matter of whether you have it or not, but whether the candida fungi exceed a normal level.

On the one hand, excessive colonization of the intestine by candida fungi is a sign of weakened body defenses. If the defenses are weakened, then the fungus has the potential to spread far too widely.

However, it is also possible that the body uses the fungi to protect itself from certain conditions such as heavy metal poisoning. Normally, the body cannot find any suitable way to rid itself of heavy metals. Therefore, its only alternative is to protect itself as much as possible from the consequences of heavy metal toxicity. It does this by binding the heavy metals to the candida fungi. At the same time, the metabolic products of candida albicans represent a lesser evil for the body than heavy metal toxicity.

Candida can spread very easily in the intestine, especially after treatment with antibiotics. Antibiotics can throw the intestinal flora out of balance and this sets up excellent living conditions for the fungus. Nevertheless, the symptoms can have a different appearance in every person: From severe flatulence, allergies and headaches to diarrhea and much more. A typical symptom of too-high candida concentration is extreme fatigue occurring sometime after eating, especially after meals that contain carbohydrates or sugars.

The reason for this is that candida fungus feeds on carbohydrates and, like most people, candida fungus loves sugar. With enough to eat, the fungus can double its population within a short time. In view of this rapid growth, the body becomes overloaded with candida metabolic products and this usually leads to this extreme fatigue shortly after eating.

If you suspect the presence of candida fungi, it is advisable to provide about two or three stool samples. This is because the fungi hang on the intestinal wall in the form of nests and not every stool sample releases enough of the fungi to make them detectable. For all other values, such as alpha-1 antitrypsin, zonulin, etc., a single sample will already be diagnostically conclusive.

We have gone through the most important values of the stool sample now. Once you get all of these laboratory values checked, you will have a clear and complete overview of what is going on in your intestine. This is already one part of your search for the cause.

In the next chapter, we will immerse ourselves deeper in the topic of the causes and discover more and more pieces of the whole puzzle about what causes digestive disorders.

Info-Box

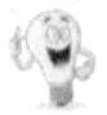

- ✓ The diagnosis always has to come first before treatment begins
- ✓ One of the best ways to find the cause of IBS is to take a stool sample
- ✓ Multiple values should be determined with a stool sample to get an overall picture of the state of the intestine

2 The causes: Where does IBS come from?

A disease is not always a bad thing – it can be more a kind of secret message from the body. Our body would like to tell us something, but the problem is that it doesn't speak our language. Instead, the body encrypts its message and speaks through the symptoms such as abdominal pain, diarrhea, a headache and so on. In order to achieve a cure for IBS and for other diseases as well, we need to understand exactly what our body wants to tell us with these symptoms. The goal is not only to suppress the symptoms, but above all to find the underlying cause. Therefore, you need to understand what your body is trying to tell you.

A headache is a great example of the language of the body. Like other pains, a headache also occurs when a signal transmitter docks on a nerve end and transmits a pain message to the brain: Attention, something is wrong here [3]. This is done via the messenger substance prostaglandin. In some cases, you take a headache pill and the pain disappears. But what does this tablet actually do? It ensures that no more messenger substances are formed – it therefore only switches the message-bearer off. Yet it does nothing to change the actual reason why the headache developed.

Let us assume that the headache was caused by a lack of fluids, simply because you drank too little throughout the day. Here, the pain is the bearer of the message "there is a lack of water." This is the body´s way of showing that there is a problem and it should be remedied. The headache tablet just switches off the pain. The message "pain" is not delivered anymore, but this does nothing to remedy the lack of fluid. If you had interpreted the pain correctly, then you would have simply solved the problem by drinking a few glasses of water.

This is the same situation as that of a king in a desert land who has to govern many cities. Of course, the king cannot be everywhere and therefore he needs messengers. One day a messenger comes by and reports to the king that at present there is a lack of water in a city of his kingdom. The king then has the messenger arrested so he won't have to be bothered with such bad news anymore. However, the water shortage continues in the city. Since the king has switched off the messenger, he no longer learns anything about the situation in that city.

The king lives on, relaxed, because there are no more bad messages bothering him and he doesn't have to worry anymore. In the afflicted city, however, the water shortage keeps getting worse. And one day the king is suddenly taken by surprise by the angry city dwellers. If the king had gotten to the root of the problem right away by taking care of the water shortage in the city, the messenger would not have come again and the king would have been spared the city dwellers' rebellion.

Now, let's transfer this example of the king to IBS. We ourselves are the king and the messengers come to us with news. This news is encoded by using the language of symptoms, such as abdominal pain, bloating, diarrhea and much more. But what is really behind the news; what does the body want to tell us?

This question about the underlying cause is always the central issue for treatment. It is of no use to just concentrate on the symptoms, for example, by taking tablets that deal with these symptoms. It is decisive to **find the cause.** You can take pills for flatulence, diarrhea or abdominal pain all your life long, but these symptoms keep on coming back nevertheless. On the other hand, you could treat the cause and the symptoms disappear on their own.

Anyone who has understood the difference between the symptoms and the causes of IBS, is someone who has already taken the most difficult step towards healing. This whole concept might sound very simple and logical, but unfortunately there are way too many doctors out there who are just focusing on suppressing the symptoms and patients have to be treated over years and years without any progress.

In the following, we will take a closer look at every single cause for IBS:

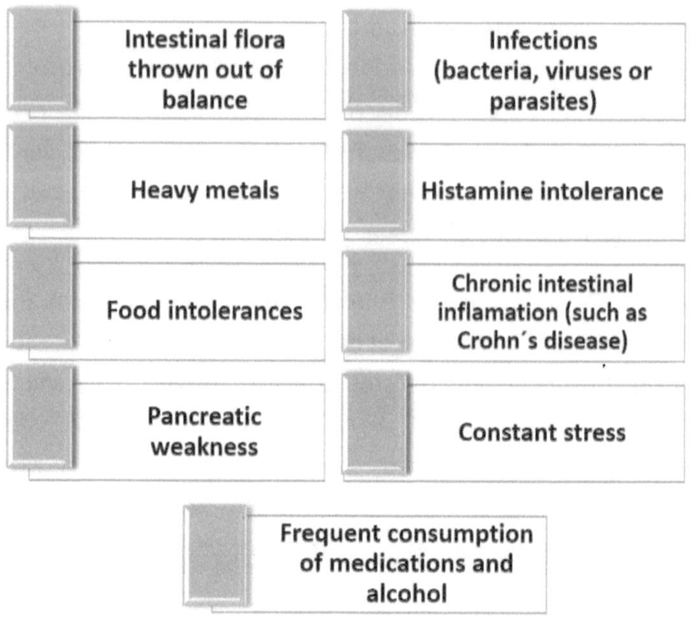

Intestinal flora: Good and bad bacteria

The intestinal flora is thrown out of balance when there are too many "bad" bacteria in the intestine and the "good" bacteria are repressed. This imbalance in the bacterial world can be triggered by the widest variety of events. One very common reason for this is taking antibiotics.

Antibiotics are administered when you have a disease caused by bacteria, such as bronchitis, or for urinary tract infections. The antibiotic simply kills the bacteria that causes the disease. In medical history, the invention of antibiotics were a huge step and antibiotics can be an absolute lifesaver.

Unfortunately, the antibiotic is not only directed against the "bad" intruder alone, but rather it also reduces the "good" bacteria in the intestine by a certain amount. Sometimes the intestinal flora will get back into balance on its own after a course of antibiotics. However, there are also many cases where digestive problems only got started after taking antibiotics. The solution here would be to take antibiotics with care and the side effects should be considered.

Besides antibiotics, a disturbed intestinal flora can also be caused by taking medications for a prolonged time, poor eating habits, preservatives, frequent use of laxatives or inflammation of the intestine.

The good bacteria ensure that the intestinal mucous membrane is constantly being regenerated. When the intestinal flora is disturbed, the mucous membrane can no longer fully bring its protective effect to bear. The result is that its protective barrier is missing and the intestine is much more exposed to toxins [4].

Usually, the "good" bacteria in the gut fights harmful invaders. However, a lack of "good" bacteria makes it much easier for intruders and harmful bacteria as well as fungi will keep spreading. Furthermore, the intestinal mucous membrane, which is like a castle wall, is thinner because of the lack of good bacteria.

Besides this, having good bacteria is extremely important for our digestion and immune system. So, there is a wide range of good reasons to check on your intestinal bacteria and to do a lot in everyday life to make them feel at home.

Infections

Infections with certain bacteria or viruses can likewise cause a severe imbalance in the intestine. Such intestinal infections include salmonella, lamblia, campylobacter, various worms, noroviruses and many more. It is easy for your therapist to check for the presence of such an infection by taking a stool and blood sample. If the findings are abnormal, the doctor then determines how to proceed with the treatment. Even though we have recognized antibiotics as a possible trigger for IBS, treatment with antibiotics can be useful if such an infection is present.

With antibiotics, the dose makes the poison: If antibiotics are used very rarely and carefully, the benefits outweigh the harm. Unfortunately, antibiotics were prescribed all too often, especially in the 1980s and 1990s, even for the mildest colds. Meanwhile, the risks of antibiotics have become better known and most doctors are much more cautious about prescribing them nowadays.

Heavy metals

Heavy metals can be another trigger of IBS. The whole issue of heavy metals is still being discussed as something very controversial in science. Some doctors still consider heavy metals to be completely harmless. By contrast, many environmental physicians strongly warn about heavy metal toxicity. As a patient, you are naturally caught between the two sides and you might ask yourself: What is it now – are heavy metals dangerous or not?

The history of amalgam fillings is a good example for this. Over the past few decades, dentists used amalgam fillings very often because they are very inexpensive and durable. Amalgam consists, among other substances, of the heavy metal mercury. These mercury fillings were considered to be completely harmless. Almost everyone who doubted or even refuted this thesis was frequently branded as a conspiracy theorist.

In the meantime, however, there has been a definite change and more and more dentists are critical of amalgam fillings. This change is evident from the fact that amalgam fillings are no longer offered in many dental practices.

In fact, it is not just that amalgam has simply been replaced nowadays because other fillers have become available. There have already been good alternatives for a long time. The change in using amalgam fillings only started because the evidence about the toxicity of this heavy metal was overwhelming. And just as even small quantities of mercury in your mouth can have massive health consequences, other heavy metals in the body also pose a significant health risk.

Environmental physicians have provided scientific evidence of the toxicity of heavy metals on many occasions [5]. Besides this, there are countless testimonials from intestinal disease patients who only were able to rid themselves of their digestive problems by having the heavy metals removed.

If you would like to have your existing amalgam fillings removed, this should only be done under strict safety precautions. These include gum shields for the teeth, special removal by suction to prevent mercury vapor, removal of the amalgam in pieces (instead by drilling) and many more. The amalgam removal therefore should only be done in any case by a specialized dentist who is experienced in this field.

The effects of heavy metals are so toxic because they can disturb many basic processes in our body. They hinder cell metabolism, change protein structures as well as enzyme functions and they can disturb detoxification.

All of these negative effects occur on a very deep cellular level. That's why heavy metals can trigger so many different diseases! You don't have to have huge amounts of mercury, aluminum or lead in your body: Even the smallest amounts in the milligram range can have serious consequences already.

One heavy metal alone can already cause serious problems. However, if there are several heavy metals in the body at the same time, their harmful effects are multiplied and they reinforce each other. Thus, one heavy metal plus one heavy metal no longer results in two possible health effects. The equation rather becomes 1 + 1 = 1,000!

Of course, every person is carrying a certain amount of heavy metals around with them and you don't always get sick from them. The decisive thing is not whether there are heavy metals in your body or not, but whether the body can still tolerate the current amount. Environmental physicians can calculate the maximum values for every single heavy metal. Up to this value, the toxicity seems to be tolerable for the majority of people.

If two or more metals exceed the respective limit, then it is no longer possible to predict the consequences at all, since they can mutually reinforce each other. Moreover, some people are very sensitive and they might react to even small amounts of heavy metals which are stored in their body.

Imagine locking a cat into a china shop alone at night. Let´s say the cat symbolizes the heavy metal mercury here. Through the night, probably just one or two vases will be broken at most; otherwise, the cat will elegantly twine itself around the porcelain. When you lock a dog into the china shop alone at night, it will sleep all night long or wait patiently for its owner. It will perhaps break just one vase as well. Let's say that the dog here stands for the heavy metal lead.

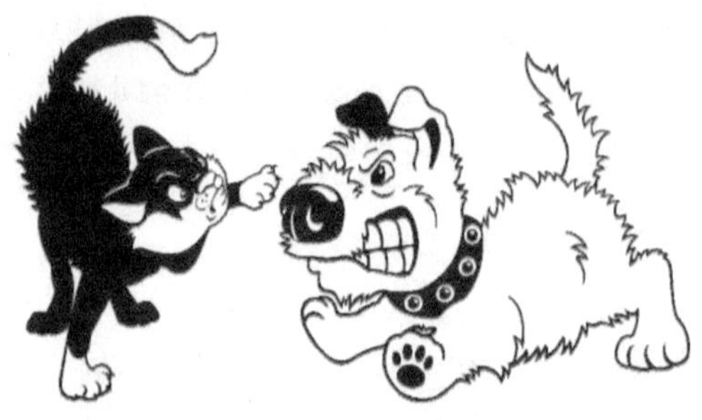

Now lock the dog and cat (mercury + lead) together in the china shop at night – the next morning you will find a lot more than just two broken vases. Both were quite peaceful on their own, but with both of them together, it is no longer possible to predict how much damage will be done to the china shop. The same is true for heavy metals in the body when there are several present at the same time.

Histamine intolerance

Histamine is a biogenic amine that is found both in food and completely naturally in our cells. If a person has histamine intolerance, the body can no longer sufficiently break down the histamine from food. The symptoms can be very different and include itching skin, facial reddening, headaches and many others.

In addition to the symptoms that you can directly notice, the excess histamine can cause further harm. We'll take a closer look at what foods contain histamine in *Chapter 3.4 Histamine: Tiny hormones with a lot of power.*

The interesting question here is: How can histamine intolerance lead to IBS? Histamine is known as an inflammatory mediator. This means that it can cause a new inflammation or it can reinforce an already existing one. Since an inflammation makes the intestine permeable, histamine intolerance can lead to the development of all kinds of a digestive disorders.

Conversely, it may also be the case that the digestive problem is present first and this leads to a more intense release of histamine. The mast cells that produce histamine are located in the connective tissue under the intestinal mucosa. If various substances that do not belong there penetrate the holey intestinal wall, one of the body's first reactions is to release histamine. The food consumed does not have to contain a lot of histamine for this to occur. The body´s own histamine can be released simply due to an ailing intestine and the release of histamine is the body's subsequently defensive reaction against the penetrating substances.

Now, we will put this information together into the puzzle and see that histamine and IBS can even cause each other. If IBS is present, more and more histamine is released in the body, since the body will defend itself against the intruders which are "slipping through." The released histamine in turn makes the inflammation in the intestine worse, because histamine is an inflammatory mediator.

These inflammatory processes exacerbate IBS and therefore more and more toxins get through the intestinal wall, which forces the body to intensify the release of histamine. This is a perfect cycle; the histamine and IBS goad each other on. The cycle starts all over again from the beginning and at the same time it keeps going all by itself!

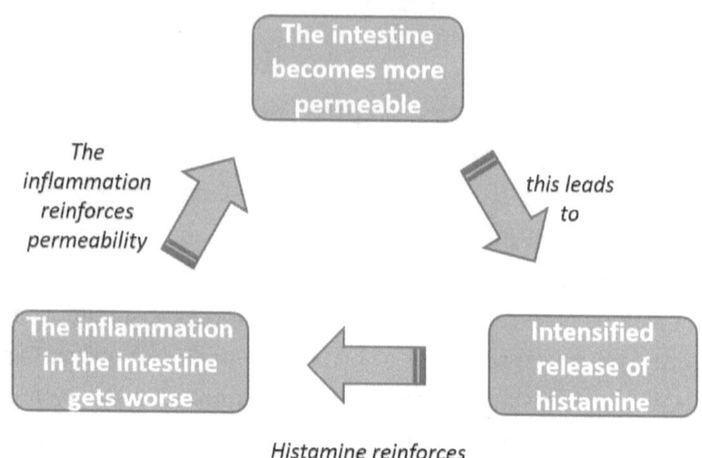

This cycle might look a little frustrating, but you shouldn´t throw in the towel out of sheer frustration. I will anticipate things at this point already: It is definitely possible to break this cycle. The most important step for you is to check if you have histamine intolerance. Nothing is worse than having histamine intolerance but you continue eating as if nothing is wrong.

Food intolerances

The Bible verse "Give us today our daily bread" shows how important consuming food is for people. If you are gluten intolerant, then daily bread would not be a good idea. The same applies if you eat certain food in spite of an intolerance. This will only cause more and more bowel irritation.

In addition to gluten intolerance, all other intolerances, such as for fructose, lactose or histamine, can have a negative effect on IBS as well. To see this connection more clearly, we will take a closer look at the lactose intolerance. Milk sugar comprises two individual sugars, glucose and galactose. These two individual sugars are closely joined together when you consume dairy products. To make it possible for the body to transfer these sugars into the blood, the bond must be broken down into the two individual sugars. This is done by the enzyme "lactase" in the intestine.

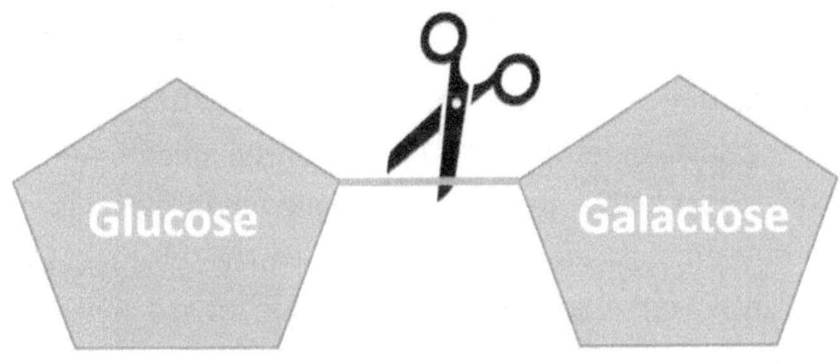

In case of lactose intolerance, this enzyme is lacking or only very little is produced. When the milk sugar is not broken down, it remains in its chain form and cannot be absorbed by the small intestine. It subsequently moves undigested into the large intestine. There the colon bacteria take care of breaking it down. However, since the large intestine is not intended to take care of this digestion step, the process is accompanied by the formation of a lot of gas and water retention – which leads to the typical symptoms of lactose intolerance: Bloating and diarrhea.

As we have seen with the example of lactose intolerance, certain types of food intolerances can cause many intestinal problems. If you continue to eat foods you cannot tolerate, they will irritate the intestine and the problem will not settle down. Therefore, it is very important to know which foods you cannot tolerate and then adjust your diet accordingly.

Chronic inflammation: Crohn's disease and ulcerative colitis

Inflammation is usually a sign that the body has to defend itself against something. The body uses the inflammation so that the respective area will be supplied with more oxygen and nutrients. At the same time, the waste substances can be transported away more quickly due to the enhanced blood flow.

Normally, an inflammation only persists until the intruder has been successfully combated and the acute condition is gone. However, sometimes the inflammation in the intestine remains permanently and over time it becomes chronic. A chronic inflammation is a sign that the cause of the inflammation is still present and the body is still actively fighting it. Another reason for the emergence of a chronic inflammation could be an imbalance of the bacteria in the intestine.

The most common forms of chronic inflammation in the intestine are Crohn's disease and ulcerative colitis. While Crohn's disease can occur in the entire digestive tract and the entire intestinal wall is inflamed, in ulcerative colitis the inflammation is just limited to the mucous membrane and only occurs in the large intestine.

If you want to rule out the presence of chronic inflammatory bowel disease, there are several options:

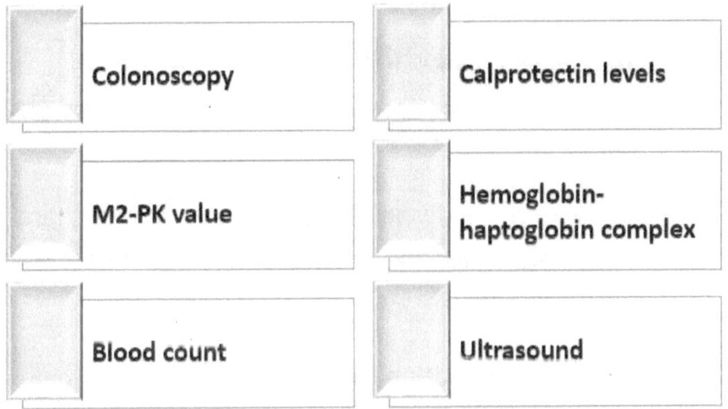

Since the symptoms appear similar in chronic inflammatory bowel disease and IBS, both diseases appear to be quite similar at first glance. Nevertheless, there are good ways to clearly differentiate between these two diseases. In case of Crohn's disease or ulcerative colitis, the mentioned laboratory values like M2-PK or hemoglobin-haptoglobin-complex are often elevated or a colonoscopy has abnormal results.

In case of IBS, these values and a colonoscopy are usually in order. A colonoscopy as well as getting the laboratory values checked can either be performed by a gastroenterologist or by a general practitioner.

Besides the laboratory values, IBS can usually be differentiated from Crohn's disease or ulcerative colitis by its symptoms:

1) With chronic inflammation, the symptoms can occur at night; with IBS the symptoms very rarely show up at night
2) IBS usually does not cause any fever, while the chronic inflammations on the other hand can cause fever
3) With Crohn's disease or ulcerative colitis there is often visible blood in the stool, but this almost never occurs with IBS

For a chronic inflammation disease, the focus is on healing the inflamed intestine (see *chapter 3.1 Good remedies against inflammation)*. The intestine does not let itself become inflamed just for fun or for no reason; there is always a cause behind the inflammation. It just takes a good diagnosis to find this cause.

Pancreatic weakness

IBS is mainly a disease of the intestine. However, if you go into the question of what led to this disease, you sometimes have to look beyond the intestine. There are multiple organs involved in the digestive chain: The stomach, the gall bladder and then the pancreas. The intestine is just the last link in the digestive chain and it has to suffer the consequences if the digestive organs that come before are not working properly.

The pancreas in particular is of enormous importance for digestion, because it forms enzymes that break down proteins, carbohydrates and fats. However, if the pancreas is not working at 100% capacity, then badly digested food will get into the intestine and it has to deal with it in addition to its normal digestive tasks.

In this case, the intestine has to take on the tasks of the pancreas. The poorly broken-down food components irritate the intestine and can lead to inflammation or growth of bad bacteria. It can also happen that portions of the badly digested food are recognized as an "enemy" and thus provoke an immune system reaction. In the long term, this overloading of the intestine will not do any good.

The pancreas is a very sensitive organ. Therefore, it may be the case that it isn't working optimally due to frequent consumption of alcohol or medications, due to stress or hyperacidity in the body. The pancreas is very sensitive to an unhealthy lifestyle and when it thinks this is too much, it goes on strike. But the pancreas isn't striking loudly and shrilly with whistles or little signs. A pancreas strike is done very quietly and silently, without you noticing it immediately.

Pancreatic weakness should not be confused with pancreatitis or the like. In case of pancreatic weakness, as the name suggests, the organ is simply weakened and by using specific remedies, it can be brought back up to speed.

You can also think of a weakness of the pancreas as something similar to having a clogged strainer on a water tap. The water (= the pancreatic secretion) then only drips out very slowly. The tap itself is fine. All you have to do is clean the strainer and the water can flow properly again.

Stress

To understand the impact of stress on the intestine, we have to look a little further back in human history. We actually have to look very far back, namely to the Stone Age. Our body has enormous potential to adapt to external circumstances and none other than Charles Darwin recognized this already in the mid-19th century: "It is not the strongest of the species that survives, nor the most intelligent that survives. It is the one that is most adaptable to change." However, this adaption takes time and our bodies still function to a very large extent just as they did during the Stone Age. Unfortunately, nowadays we are very often at the mercy of everyday stress and this combination of a "Stone Age body" with modern permanent stress can lead to many diseases.

In a calm environment, our intestine is constantly busy with digestion and it uses quite a lot of energy to accomplish this. If a saber-toothed tiger suddenly jumps out of the bushes, the body has to switch to an attack or escape mode at lightning speed. It must have a lot of energy available within seconds. The time of calm and relaxed digestion is over within a second. What the body needs most of all now are salts and high-energy substances. In the end, it has to be ready to immediately run away from the attacker.

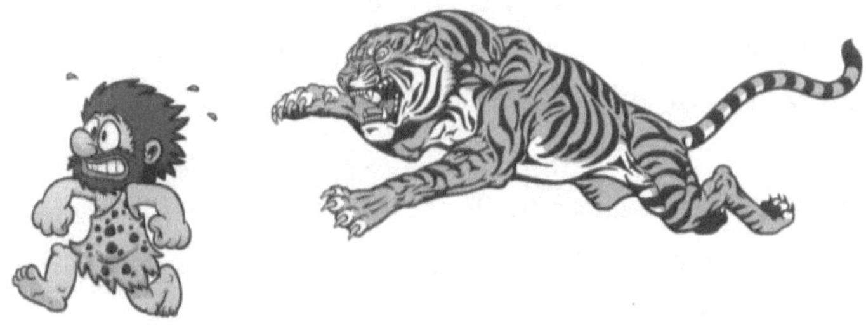

In such a situation, the protein SGLT-1 is activated to make it possible for the substances to get through the intestinal wall more quickly. This protein makes the gaps between two cells in the intestinal wall (the “tight junctions”) wider. The intestinal wall consequently becomes more permeable so that the energy-rich substances needed for fleeing are absorbed more quickly. In an extreme situation, that's a very helpful process!

If we are in this state of stress just for a short time, this isn’t critical at all. As soon as we are safe, the cell spacing in the intestine becomes tight and the body can devote itself to digesting food normally again. However, what happens when we experience daily stress as if we had to run away from a tiger every day? Then the spaces between cells remain permanently expanded and we have a classic leaky gut syndrome.

Therefore, stress can definitely be seen as an important trigger for IBS. Even if stress is something on the psychological level and IBS involves the body, the state of mind and body are very closely connected to each other. If things are not going well mentally, the body suffers. This also works the other way around: When your body is in pain or you struggle with any other physical disturbances, your mind and your well-being can also be disturbed. The mind and the body are very closely connected to each other and when one suffers, the other one suffers as well.

Frequent consumption of medications and alcohol

As already described, antibiotics take a lot out of the good bacteria and as a result, the intestinal flora changes. However, in addition to antibiotics, prolonged use of any medication can also result in digestive disorders.

Especially **painkillers**, such as ASA (aspirin), ibuprofen, naproxen or diclofenac very often harm the intestine when they are used for a long time. They don't in fact destroy the good gut bacteria like antibiotics do, but they damage the protective intestinal mucosa. This can even go so far as causing internal bleeding. That is why in Germany, the statutory health insurance companies have to spend tens of millions each year to treat the secondary diseases caused by the effects of medications on the stomach and intestine.

Once the protective intestinal mucosa has been weakened, the intestine is helplessly exposed to the invading viruses, parasites or harmful bacteria. Since the intestinal mucosa has been impaired by the medication and no longer offers full protection against intruders, the intestine can only fight back by means of an inflammatory reaction.

In just the same way as certain medications do, frequent alcohol consumption also impairs the intestinal mucosa. If the intestine is permeable and you still consume a lot of alcohol, then the toxic substances from the alcohol are able to get into the body unhindered and cause further harm.

Unfortunately, excessive alcohol consumption is not uncommon at all. There are around 1.77 million alcoholics just in Germany alone, and about 200 people die every day (!) from the consequences of their risky alcohol consumption. The treatment of alcohol-related diseases costs some 27 billion euros every year [6].

Nevertheless, we shouldn't get carried away with the issue of alcohol too much: A glass now and then will by no means cause digestive disorders. Only the daily consumption of larger amounts is very critical, because the body does not get any time to regenerate itself.

Info-Box 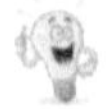

- ✓ It usually isn't possible to determine the exact cause of IBS just by the symptoms
- ✓ It is always decisive to treat the causes, not just to suppress the symptoms
- ✓ There can be several reasons for developing IBS: Disturbed intestinal flora, infections, heavy metal toxicity, food intolerances, histamine intolerance, stress or long term use of medications and alcohol

3 The treatment – Step by step back to a carefree life

After taking a closer look at the reasons why IBS develops, we now turn to what is likely the most exciting question: How do I get rid of my digestive disorders? The most important therapeutic measures to accomplish this are described in the following sections. The measures are presented in such a way that the most important ones come first.

The individual measures are also not mutually exclusive and several treatments can be implemented simultaneously. For example, it is possible to deal with an inflammation while improving the condition of the intestinal flora at the same time.

It is very important that you don't just take any medication indiscriminately. Here too, the old wisdom applies: "Before the treatment, the gods made the diagnosis." Therefore, you should first test for what is causing your condition in general: histamine, heavy metals, weakness of the pancreas and so on. I have listed the corresponding testing methods for every possible cause. This is the diagnostics part and it always comes first.

Only when you are certain that your values are significant, then you can proceed on to the treatment. For example, it wouldn´t make sense to fight inflammation in your intestine if your intestine isn´t even inflamed. I have to repeat myself here, because things are often done the wrong way around and this sequence is of enormous importance: First the diagnosis, then the treatment!

Food supplements work especially well for healing digestive problems. However, the question immediately arises: Where can I get food supplements that contain as few ingredients and are as natural as possible? On the one hand, you don't want to burden your body with a lot of additives. Most of the time, IBS patients cannot tolerate certain ingredients, for example if they are histamine or lactose intolerant.

Therefore, the company "Pure Encapsulations" has specialized in food supplements which contain very few additives. Since IBS patients very often have to struggle with intolerances, it is very important that they don't irritate their intestine further by consuming additives.

In addition to taking food supplements, your **everyday lifestyle** is also crucial for getting well again. It just doesn't work if you take the very best food supplements, but at the same time you don't pay attention to your health on an everyday basis. As a result, your well-intentioned efforts will fizzle out completely.

Commitment to your everyday lifestyle should embrace all areas. If you live a very healthy life by doing a lot of sports, not smoking, eating a healthy diet and also take care of your mental balance – but at the same time you drink five beers or half a bottle of whiskey every evening, things won't go well over the long term. It's also not a good idea to either overdo sports or do none at all. Just like with most things, the truth lies in the golden mean. It is better you do 80% of what is needed for every single lifestyle factor (like smoking, alcohol, healthy eating, exercise) but at the same time you don't forget any one of them.

The issue of having a healthy lifestyle is present everywhere: On TV, in magazines or at school. You might already get annoyed about the hundredth time you are given a tip on how you should always be very disciplined. However, when you are struggling with severe digestive problems, it is extremely helpful to take a closer look at your daily lifestyle and to keep on improving it. Your body will be happy about any help you can offer it! In my own experience, changing little things in everyday life and listening very carefully to your body´s messages is one of the best therapies.

Keep in mind that when your intestine is already weakened, it will of course have a much more sensitive reaction to most external influences than a healthy intestine will. Once the intestine is better, you can relax this "strict" lifestyle a bit more.

The most important lifestyle factors are once again summarized in brief in the following. Even if it is already well known: All of these factors have a major impact on IBS and on your health in general:

No alcohol
Healthy food
No smoking
Avoid stress
Plenty of exercise
Good night´s sleep

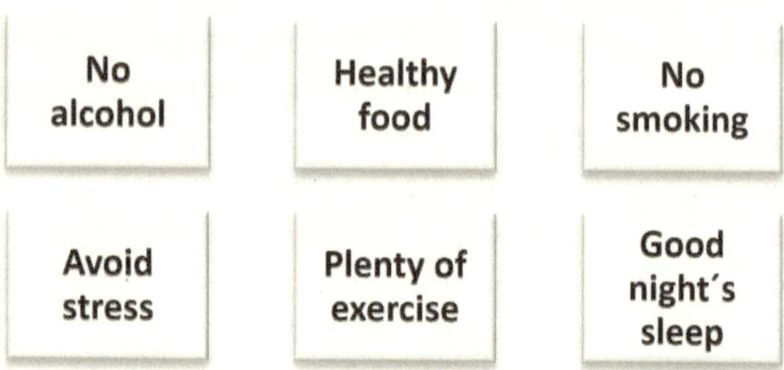

It is hard work to change something in your lifestyle. If it were easy, you would have probably changed it already, especially if you have habits that you've grown fond of over many years. In contrast, it is significantly easier to just swallow a tablet and have the good sensation that you are "doing something for your health."

A healthy lifestyle might sound too simple, but even the best tablets don't make up for a bad lifestyle. Here you have to literally swallow a bitter pill. If you want to do things the right way, a good lifestyle goes hand in hand with structured treatment to heal your digestive problems.

3.1 Good remedies against inflammation

Many digestive disorders involve inflammation. Due to the inflammation, the distance between the cells in the intestinal mucous membrane increases and the intestine becomes permeable. It also works the other way around – the intestine can be permeable first and this causes the inflammation. The question of whether the chicken (permeability) or the egg (inflammation) came first can be left to the philosophers. For us, this plays no role in any further approach and we are rather focusing on the healing process.

The big problem is that the inflammation and the permeability mutually reinforce each other, just like in our example of the dog and the cat in the china shop. When the intestine is permeable, then inflammation occurs. This inflammation then causes the intestine to become even more permeable, which in turn leads to an even worse inflammation ... and the cycle starts all over again.

Sometimes, whatever it is that triggered the digestive problems has already disappeared, but the cycle of permeability and inflammation keeps on going all by itself. At this point, the crucial thing is to break the cycle and the best way to achieve this is using remedies that have an anti-inflammatory effect.

How is inflammation in the intestine measured?
The most uncomplicated and reliable method for checking for the presence of inflammation is a stool sample. To do this, a natural practitioner or doctor simply sends your stool sample to a laboratory and you get the results within a few days. Based on the **alpha-1 antitrypsin** as well as the **calprotectin** values, it is possible to recognize whether inflammation is present in the intestine or not.

Besides these two values, you should take the opportunity and have other values measured as well. Even if it costs a little more, there can be many causes for an intestinal problem and it isn't possible to discover it just from one or two laboratory values. At the same time, it is fascinating that science nowadays is so advanced that it can learn so much about our intestine from just a single stool sample.

What can I do about the inflammation?
First the good news: If the stool analysis demonstrates that there is inflammation present in your intestine, there is a great deal that can be done about it. Here, we are not just talking about artificially suppressing the inflammation with cortisone, because administering cortisone has far too many side effects in the long run. The goal is to provide the body with many helpful nutrients and supplements so that it can heal the inflammation on its own.

Vitamin C is a highly effective anti-inflammatory agent. Free radicals are generated especially by inflammation processes. These free radicals are not some kind of hooligans running wild, but rather they are oxygen compounds that protect you from intruders or eliminate cells that have died. However, if there are too many free radicals present in your body, then this will damage cells as well as tissues and the inflammation will become more intense.

Radical scavengers like vitamin C are also known as antioxidants. They work very well for fighting an inflammation. However, you have to be aware that even a healthy body needs a certain quantity of vitamin C for its everyday processes.

At the end of the day, even if you eat a healthy diet, there is usually not much additional vitamin C left in your body which will help to fight the inflammation. This is why it is necessary to consume significantly larger quantities of vitamin C than a healthy person does, since it is needed for everyday processes and additionally for fighting the inflammation.

The good thing about taking vitamin C: You can take it in larger amounts. Since it is a water-soluble vitamin, the body can simply excrete excess quantities in the urine. For guidance, the German Nutrition Society recommends about 100 mg of vitamin C per day for healthy people [7]. If there is an inflammation in the intestine, the daily intake should therefore be a lot higher.

Usually, it is not possible to ensure you get this necessary amount by eating a healthy diet. Just to consume enough to obtain 300 mg, which is 300% of the daily value, you would have to eat six oranges or lemons every day. In terms of taste, this would already be a top accomplishment, but eating this huge number of oranges is not a good idea at all for a damaged intestine. That is why it makes sense to rely on food supplements at this point.

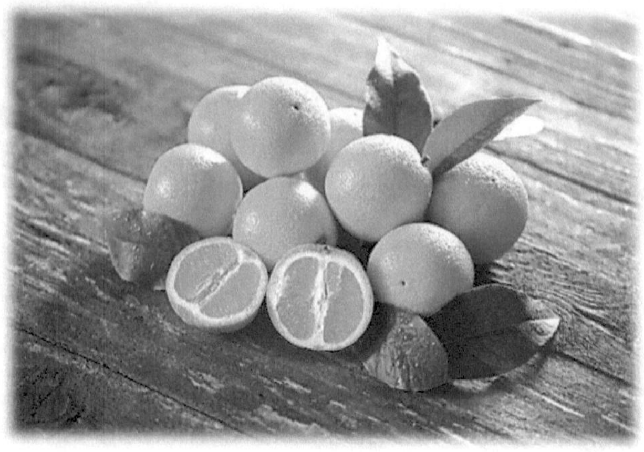

Most supplements come in the form of powders or tablets. However, the full quantity stated on the package does not end up in your body, because a certain quantity is always lost in the digestive process.

A **high-dose infusion of vitamin C,** on the other hand, works differently. This method can administer 10 to 20 grams (not milligrams!) with a single infusion. This corresponds to 10,000 to 20,000 mg or about 400 lemons at one time. At the same time, the body can use 100% of this quantity, since it is available directly in the blood and does not have to travel through the entire digestive tract. The only downside is the cost of a high-dose infusion. In comparison, food supplements are significantly less expensive. With the right preparation, however, the costs are not a problem. There is more about how to cover the costs in *Chapter 5*.

The medical terms for inflammation are quite interesting. Disease names associated with inflammation often end with *–itis*, for example, arthr*itis* (joint inflammation), dermat*itis* (skin inflammation) or gastr*itis* (stomach inflammation).

Besides vitamin C, **amino acids** also work very well for fighting inflammation. When you consume protein along with your food, it is not possible for the intestine to simply absorb it right away into the blood. This is similar to lactose, which is first broken down into the individual sugars.

Protein must likewise be broken down into smaller units. These smaller parts are called amino acids. The intestine is only able to absorb these amino acids, transfer them to the blood and then use them for various processes in the body. However, there are certain products to buy that contain protein which has already been broken down into amino acids.

The amino acid **L-glutamine** has especially proven itself very well as a treatment against inflammation. How important L-glutamine is for the intestine, is shown by the fact that around 40% of total glutamine consumption takes place only in the intestine [8]. This is because L-glutamine can reduce the permeability of the intestinal mucous membrane and alleviate inflammatory processes, and these are exactly the two positive effects which you need.

The intestinal mucous membrane is made up of cells that divide very quickly and they particularly like L-glutamine for their growth process. These cells renew themselves completely every three to four days and there is always a lot happening in the intestinal mucous membrane. Besides supporting cell recovery, L-glutamine also helps to restore the protective barrier of the small intestine mucous membrane. As we have seen before, this membrane is usually damaged when you have an inflammation.

In total, there are 21 different amino acids and they occur in a balanced relationship. Therefore, you should not take a single amino acid like L-glutamine over a longer period (maximum of six to eight weeks). If you supplement a single amino acid over a long time, it would shift the entire amino acid profile in your body and this will cause negative effects in other places.

L-glutamine can be taken as a supplement for a few weeks to support cell recovery and build up intestinal mucous membrane, but then you should take a break. The recommended dosage of L-glutamine is about 3-5 g per day. It is also crucial here that you are able to tolerate the quantity you are taking and you might want to sneak it in by starting with a small quantity and slowly increasing your intake.

As with vitamin C, amino acids can also be administered through an infusion. Some companies have even calibrated the composition of the amino acids in the infusion specifically for inflammation and leaky gut syndrome.

Next to vitamin C and L-glutamine, the trace element **zinc** is also very important for successful treatment. It has many properties that are urgently needed to deal with a permeable intestine: It supports wound healing and especially the build-up of the mucous membrane. Zinc is involved in more than 300 enzyme processes throughout the body and it has an anti-inflammatory effect, which is just what you need when you are struggling with an inflammation in the intestine.

However, when taking zinc, there are a number of things to consider so that the effects can evolve to the full extent. Certain substances like iron or folic acid hinder the absorption of zinc in the intestine [9]. Therefore, zinc should be taken at least one hour apart from meals. It is ideal to take it in the evening and in combination with vitamin C, because the vitamin C even improves the absorption of zinc. Since these two supplements are mutually reinforcing, they are called co-factors. Thus, taking vitamin C and zinc together is twice as good: Both help with inflammation and they mutually reinforce each other.

As already mentioned for vitamin C, taking a higher dosage is not so critical, since it is a water-soluble vitamin and the body can simply excrete unused quantities. On the other hand, things are very different for zinc; here you should carefully comply with the recommended dose. The German Society for Nutrition recommends around 11-16 mg zinc for adult men and 7-10 mg zinc for adult women per day [10].

Another great supplement when it comes to healing the inflammation is **bone broth** and it has become a whole new trend. In fact, it was already well known in grandma's day and it is right back in fashion and that's a good thing. There are even specialty shops in some cities that specialize in bone broth. The special thing about these shops is that they simmer the broth for more than 24 hours. The fact that bone broth is so fashionable now is not just a general fitness trend. Above all, it is because there are significantly more people who have digestive problems and this issue is of concern to more and more people now.

Bone broth is very rich in collagen and this is particularly valuable to our digestive tract. Collagen helps to rebuild the protective intestinal mucous membrane and thus to protect the intestine from unwanted intruders. Besides this, bone broth contains amino acids such as proline, glycine and gelatin – and here we are again with our amino acids, whose great effects we had already discussed before.

To benefit from the healing effects of bone broth, it is very important that it is simmered for at least three to four hours or even longer. Only then, the amino acids and collagen are released. In terms of taste, you can spice up bone broth any way you like.

If the cooking time to make bone broth takes too long for you, you can also buy ready-made bone broth. Good manufacturers have simmered the bone broth slowly for 20 hours or more and there is usually laboratory verification of the collagen content. Making the bone broth yourself is of course much less expensive, but it also takes a lot of time.

When you are suffering from an inflammation, we have already described the four "magic cures" to effectively build up the mucous membrane and to fight inflammation: Vitamin C, amino acids (especially L-glutamine), zinc and bone broth.

In addition, many other remedies for curing the inflammation have also proven their worth:

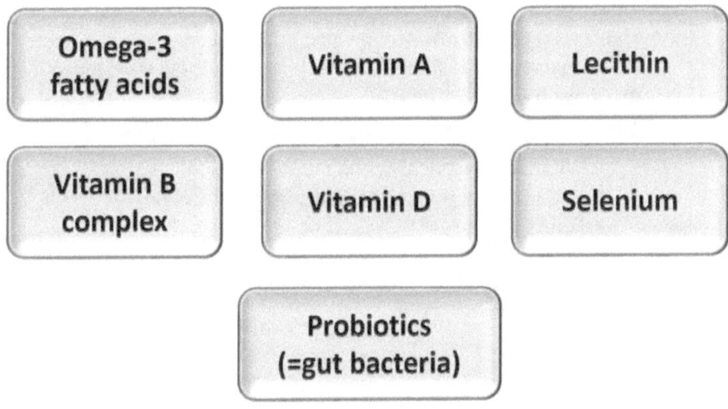

In particular, consuming sufficient quantities of **vitamin D** is really crucial. This is because this vitamin is involved in many processes and it supports the body in fighting inflammation by capturing the free radicals. Nowadays, most people have a vitamin D deficiency because we spend too much time of the day indoors. Besides staying inside too much, in northern latitudes the levels of solar radiation are low most of the year.

With modern laboratory tests, it is very easy to determine if you have a vitamin D deficiency. If your vitamin D level is low, then you can compensate for this by taking a vitamin D supplement.

Info-Box 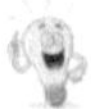

- ✓ Sometimes a self-sustaining cycle of inflammation and permeability is created
- ✓ This cycle can be broken by taking measures that are anti-inflammatory and at the same time build up the mucous membrane
- ✓ Some very good remedies are:
  - Vitamin C (especially a high-dose infusion)
  - L-Glutamine (as well as amino acids in general)
  - Zinc
  - Bone broth
  - Vitamin D level should be checked

3.2 Food intolerances

When the gut is inflamed and permeable, a very common reaction is the development of food intolerances. Here again, you can pose yourself the philosophical question: What came first – the inflammation or the food intolerance?

However, in terms of the further healing process, it doesn't matter at all what came first. At this point, it is much more important to find out which food intolerances are present and to know that eating incompatible foods can make the digestive disorders worse.

The insidious thing about food intolerances: It is very difficult at the beginning to identify which foods you tolerate well and which foods make trouble. When you eat a meal with five different ingredients and you are intolerant of just one, then you might get bloating or diarrhea only from this one intolerant ingredient. Unfortunately, there is no sign that tells you which exact food from that meal you can´t digest well. All you can do here is to carefully listen to your body.

And just so that things don't get too easy, most reactions won´t come up immediately but they are delayed, sometimes even 24 to 48 hours later. For example, if your belly starts rumbling shortly after lunch or if you suddenly experience bloating or diarrhea, then it is mostly not because of the meal you just ate. After all, the meal you just ate hasn't even left the stomach after such a short time. For example, meat can even remain in your stomach for three to five hours and it only then starts to reach the intestine slowly.

However, there are foods that cause trouble immediately after you eat them. If problems such as stomach pangs or histamine symptoms like red or itchy skin appear immediately after eating, then they are very likely caused by the meal you have just eaten. So, the time to react to a food can range from seconds up to more than one day.

As you can see, it is far from easy to find out what has triggered your digestive disorders, but the more you can narrow down what the critical foods are, the more you help your intestine to recover.

Before you start testing for food intolerances right away, you can already begin by rounding up the usual suspects. There are certain foods that are quite well known for causing problems:

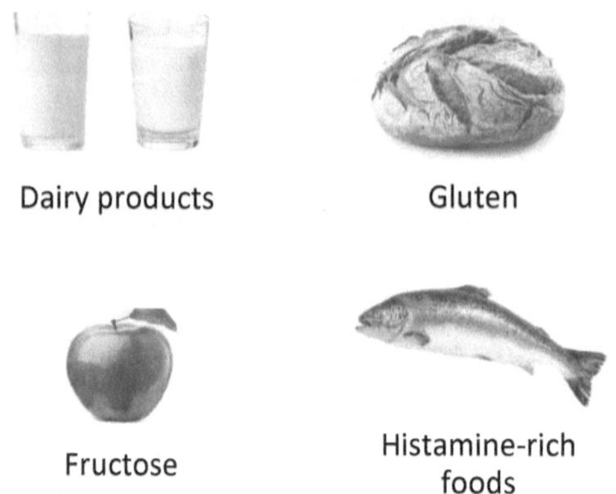

To check if you have a food intolerance, you can exclude certain foods from your meal plan – this is called an elimination diet. However, you shouldn't eliminate all foods at once; instead, you can simply test things out by excluding the foods from a certain group (dairy products, gluten, fructose or histamine) for one or two weeks. In case you are intolerant of a certain food, you should feel significantly better by omitting these food items in the phase of abstinence.

How to test for a food intolerance?

There are many different opinions about the right way to test for a food intolerance, because there are different test procedures for lactose, fructose and histamine intolerance. This makes it even more difficult for anyone affected to find a reliable test.

Unfortunately, many wheeler-dealers have already made their way into this market and are making tons of money by offering test procedures that don't work at all. We will now bring some clarity into this impenetrable jungle of test procedures, and I will show you which test procedures you can confidently omit.

Using a bad test is not only about the lost money. Moreover, when an unreliable test for an intolerance is used, the results may even be completely false. Based on this false test, it is suggested that you should no longer eat certain foods, even though your body can tolerate these foods very well. By eliminating such foods, you unnecessarily narrow down your diet without any positive effects.

But it can even get worse: An unreliable test can say that you can tolerate a food perfectly, but in fact it is exactly this food that causes the biggest trouble. Based on the test result, you think you are safe and you keep eating this food, but in fact, this makes your digestive problems even worse and the intestine gets irritated again and again. That is why good, reliable tests are so important.

Some people may secretly hope that they could measure all their possible food intolerances with just one single test. I am very sorry to be the bearer of bad news, but there is no "all-in-one" test!

Actually, there is already such a test and it is widely advertised, but I can only strongly advise against it. This test is known as the IgG antibody test. Many home self-tests also work on this principle. It can always be recognized by the designation "**IgG**." Meanwhile, associations of allergy physicians all around the world are warning about these IgG tests. For example, the German (DGAKI), Austrian (ÖGAI), Swiss (SGAI), European (EAACI), American (AAAAI) and Canadian (CSACI) associations are all criticizing this test very emphatically [11; 14].

Instead of getting this IgG test done, you might as well toss a coin: Heads you have an intolerance, tails you have none. Since this test is meanwhile being advertised very widely and many patients do not know what is behind it, we will take a closer look at the procedure.

The IgG antibody test checks whether the immune system reacts to a certain food or not. This is the really important part here: The IgG-test only looks at the immune system, nothing else! More precisely, it looks at the reaction of the **I**mmuno**g**lobulin **G** (IgG).

Let's take an example and assume that you are lactose intolerant. This means that you cannot tolerate dairy products because you produce too little or none of the enzyme lactase in your intestine. In this case, milk sugar is not digested in the small intestine, as it should be. Instead, it slips on into the large intestine and causes serious problems there. This is because the large intestine usually has nothing at all to do with digesting milk sugar.

Now, the IgG test does not measure the amount of the enzyme lactase in your body, which is in almost all cases the cause of a lactose intolerance. Instead, it only looks to see if your immune system has a reaction to dairy products, totally ignoring the amount of lactase enzyme present. You get your test result, saying that you can continue to consume dairy products without any problem.

As said before, the actual cause of lactose intolerance is that your intestine does not form enough of the enzyme lactase and therefore the milk sugar is not broken down properly in the intestine. In this case, it does not matter at all how your immune system reacts to milk: As long as you don't have enough enzymes in your intestine to break down lactose, you will still not tolerate dairy products. The IgG test therefore is making the measurement in the completely wrong place. If you continue to consume dairy products because of the false IgG-test results, the intestine becomes even more irritated and your digestive problems simply will not calm down.

I would normally not go into detail on such a misleading test at all since we want to focus on helpful, reliable tests. Unfortunately, the IgG test has meanwhile become very common, the companies involved are earning tons of money and patients are being left with completely false results.

But how can you recognize if someone offers you a good, reliable test or not? One hint is simply the number of foods that a test measures at once. Good, reliable tests can normally just measure one intolerance at a time; either it is lactose, fructose, gluten or histamine. On the other hand, an unreliable test like the IgG-test claims that it can measure around 100 foods and allergies at a time.

And it is not only in cases of lactose intolerance that the IgG-test measures incorrectly. The test also does not detect fructose intolerance at all. The transporter GLUT-5 is needed in appropriate amounts to transport fructose into the blood system. As we discussed before, the IgG test only measures the reaction of the immune system and will never really detect if you have enough of the GLUT-5 transporter.

And the same applies for histamine. In this case, the patients often lack the enzyme DAO, but the IgG test doesn't care – it happily keeps measuring only the immune system reaction. So, stay away from this quackery, because nowadays there are tests that can reliably check for food intolerances in a very scientific way.

This is not done by means of a single test, but instead there is a separate test procedure for each intolerance. The results from these tests are then very reliable:

Intolerance	Currently best testing option
Histamine intolerance	- Measure DAO value and total histamine level in blood - Elimination diet (avoid histamine)
Lactose intolerance	- Hydrogen breath test for lactose
Fructose intolerance	- Hydrogen breath test for fructose
Gluten intolerance (celiac disease)	- Blood test for: -> Transglutaminase-IgA -> Endomysium-IgA -> Total-IgA - Elimination diet (omit gluten)

Table 1: The best tests for food intolerances.

Even if it´s a bit more complex to perform the intolerance tests individually, in return you will get scientific and very reliable results. If I had to test myself for food intolerances again, I would start with the most common ones: Histamine as well as gluten both using a blood test and lactose as well as fructose both using a hydrogen breath test.

Besides testing in a laboratory, there is another simple way of checking for food intolerances and this applies for all intolerances: The least expensive and most reliable method for testing is an elimination diet. The appropriate food group (dairy products, fructose, gluten or histamine) is simply completely eliminated from the diet for about two to three weeks and the change in symptoms is noted in a nutritional record. Should your digestive problems improve significantly by eliminating a certain group of foods, then you have most likely already found the trigger of your digestive disorders.

What can you do about a food intolerance?

A food intolerance is almost always only a result of another disease and they are innate only in very rare cases. Mostly, food intolerances develop during the course of life, triggered by a certain cause. And this cause or underlying disease has to be dealt with in order to cure the intolerance.

If certain foods are causing digestive problems for you at the moment, then they have to be eliminated from your diet. The goal is to get more and more foods back on the menu over the long term. This happens when the intestine has calmed down again and when the underlying disease has been cured. Therefore, you should proceed as follows:

1) Recognize any food intolerance
2) Eliminate the food you can't tolerate from your diet
3) Cure the "underlying disease"

By the term underlying disease, I mean all the causes which are listed in *Chapter 2*, such as an imbalance in the intestinal flora, heavy metals, a weakened pancreas and many more.

In general, nutrition is an extremely important matter for people who have IBS. Even the best and most expensive treatments are of little use if you do not adjust your nutritional plan. If you have intestinal problems, then completely different eating and lifestyle principles apply than those for people with a healthy intestine.

Salads, raw foods or whole grains are often recommended for good nutrition. As someone with intestinal afflictions, you can immediately throw these recommendations overboard, because they were made for the average healthy person. If you have a damaged intestine, you should rather eat foods that are **cooked or steamed**, reduce consumption of raw foods and also lower your intake of whole grains. They strain the intestine too much and this is not helpful when your intestine is already agitated.

If you can tolerate eating raw foods or whole grains despite having digestive problems, you can of course include both on your menu in small amounts. When the therapy goes well and your intestine is feeling better again, these nutritional recommendations are great for you. However, keep in mind that they are made for healthy people and they won't be helpful for a damaged intestine at all.

Another important point is the **serving size**. Of course, it is always pleasant when food tastes good, because a delicious meal is also good for the soul. However, you should not overtax your intestine, which is already overwhelmed anyway, with serving sizes that are too large. It is better to eat several smaller servings than one very large portion.

The old saying "Eat like an emperor in the morning, like a king at noon and like a beggar in the evening," is a golden rule for anyone who has a digestive disorder. Especially the time lapse between dinner and bedtime is crucial and should be at least four hours. If you eat late in the evening and then go straight to bed, the body switches to sleep mode and no longer digests the food properly. In the end, it is our dear intestine that suffers the consequences!

Right at the beginning, it is really difficult to recognize which foods should be avoided. Especially when you are affected by several intolerances at the same time, it quickly becomes confusing trying to figure out what you can still eat. However, it has been shown that certain foods are very digestible and they can help you to calm down your digestive system. These include:

Rice (not whole grain)	**Gluten-free noodles (not whole grain)**
Potatoes (peeled)	**Millet/ buckwheat (not whole grain)**
Butter	**Vegetables (cooked)**

To get a better overview in the jungle of recipes and foods, a nutritional consultation can also be a very useful addition. You can often get many good tips from the nutritionist and some health insurers will even cover these costs.

Nevertheless, we don't just want to stop at how you should avoid certain foods for the rest of your life and how to live with a restricted diet. Rather, we now want to go more deeply into the root causes of IBS.

3.3 Pep up your intestinal flora

Already in the 16th century, the gifted physician Paracelsus coined the phrase "Death sits in the intestine." Also, Hippocrates discovered in 300 BC that "a bad digestion is the root of all evil." A sick intestine can thus be responsible for many different diseases. Even for symptoms that at first glance have nothing at all to do directly with digestion, such as headaches, skin problems, fatigue, joint problems and so on. The position of the intestine in the body is very central and this shows already that it plays a central role for good health.

This interrelationship between the intestine and overall health is even more obvious for someone with IBS. When the intestine is permeable, a lot more toxins get into the body than when the intestine is healthy and this can result in the most diverse range of diseases throughout the entire body.

As we have already seen, too many "bad" bacteria in the gut can be the cause for digestive disorders. There are a lot of possible reasons why the intestinal flora might be out of balance. One thing that the intestinal flora does not like at all are antibiotics. The word “anti” means against and "bios" means life. Already from the meaning of the word antibiotics, it quickly becomes clear that these drugs are "against life." More specifically, they are directed against bacteria.

This can be a life-saver in case of very serious diseases, but too frequent use makes the intestinal flora suffer. The antibiotic doesn’t just locate and kill the "bad" bacteria. Rather, an antibiotic takes action against a specific spectrum of bacteria. Unfortunately, while it is fighting the intruders, it also destroys a certain number of "good" bacteria. In some cases, the intestine can recover on its own after you take antibiotics. However, sometimes the recovery just doesn't work on its own and the intestinal gut flora will remain imbalanced!

If too many "good" gut bacteria have been destroyed, then harmful bacteria will spread very quickly in the intestine, because there are no opponents to the “bad” bacteria which ensure law and order. The harmful bacteria produce toxins and they attack the intestinal mucous membrane. Due to the lack of good gut bacteria, new invaders have an easier time and the intestinal mucous membrane is helplessly exposed to these attacks.

This state of things can be readily compared to that of a medieval castle. The "good" gut bacteria are the castle inhabitants who have built a thick wall around the castle for protection. If there are too few castle inhabitants to defend it, then the attackers have it easy. They pierce holes in the castle wall (here, meaning in the intestinal mucous membrane) to get into the castle. Since there are too few castle inhabitants, they can no longer protect the castle wall.

Once the intruders make it through the protective wall, they force the castle inhabitants back. Since the protective wall is now "holey," more and more attackers keep following. Only when there are enough castle inhabitants to build up the protective wall again, it is then possible to stop the attack and recapture the castle.

Nevertheless, it is not just antibiotics that can seriously throw the intestinal flora out of balance. Preservatives can kill off the good gut bacteria as well. They are made to store food and beverages over a longer time by killing or slowing down the growth process of fungi and bacteria. Unfortunately, this process does not just work in a jar, but also in our intestine.

Another bad factor for our gut bacteria is consistent poor nutrition, because the "bad" bacteria in our intestine love sugar and white flour. If they are constantly being resupplied, they multiply splendidly and force the "good" gut bacteria further and further back. Conversely, a healthy diet is a great nutritional base for the good gut bacteria, because they love vegetables and fiber. However, if you have an intolerance you should only consume foods which you can tolerate well.

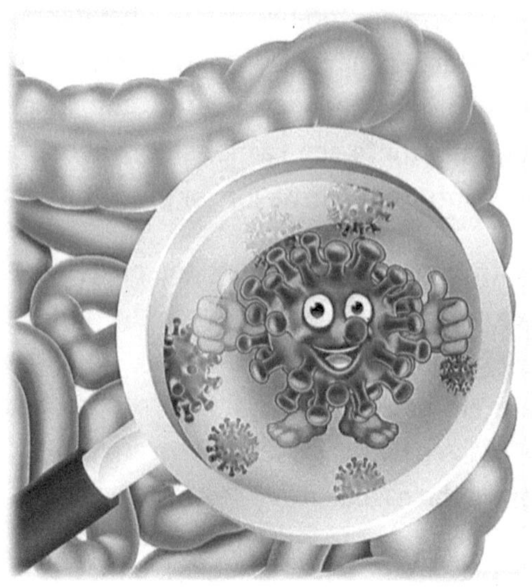

The constant use of disinfectants also has negative consequences for our intestine. If you are constantly disinfecting all surfaces and your hands, then the immune system will hardly be challenged. Once the immune system does have to deal with germs and bacteria again, then it is usually quickly overwhelmed. A good balanced level of hygiene is very important, but excessive hygiene can lead to more problems than benefits in the long term.

How do you measure gut bacteria?

A stool sample works very well for checking the condition of the intestinal flora. At the same time, it is possible to determine both the number of "good" bacteria and the number of most "bad" bacteria.

The pH value in the intestine also has a big impact on the intestinal flora. Once again, this pH value in the intestine is something different from the pH value in the urine, which is used to measure the general over-acidification of the body. The intestinal pH level should move in the range from 5.8 to 6.5. The "bad" bacteria feel particularly well at a pH value above 6.5 and spread much faster. This pH value can also be determined from a stool sample.

However, there are more factors, besides a lack of good gut bacteria or a bad pH value, that can be responsible for digestive problems. It is also possible that a viral infection, bacterial pathogens or worms are responsible for the digestive problems. These intruders can likewise cause problems and ultimately lead to IBS. Science has developed very far in this area, and it has meanwhile become possible to identify many pests through laboratory tests.

To get an examination for viruses, pathogens or worms, you should ask your general practitioner or a gastroenterologist about it. The following overview serves as a small guide to the things the doctor can test for in association with intestinal and digestive problems:

Viruses
such as adeno- ,astro-, rota- or norovirus

Bacteria
such as campylobacter, salmonella, shigella or yersinia

Protozoans
such as amoebas, lamblia or cryptosporidium

Worms
and worm eggs

Fungi
such as candida

You can already see from the list of intruders that the intestine is constantly threatened from many sides. The good news is that testing is very easy and a variety of pests can be identified by means of a single blood or stool sample.

What can you do to improve your intestinal flora?

Before we deal with how we can reintroduce good gut bacteria, we first have to create the appropriate basic conditions for the bacteria. If you take probiotics, you naturally want many of the good bacteria to settle in your intestine and remain "living" there. In fact, just as we are picky when it comes to choosing a nice home, gut bacteria also choose their living environment very carefully and want it to be cozy.

The intestinal pH value is particularly important for making sure that your gut bacteria really feel well. If the pH value is higher than 6.5, the intestinal flora can be acidified with lactic acid (so called "L+" products). Lactic acid is available in pharmacies and you can use it to already furnish the gut bacteria's home beautifully, so that they feel as 'snug as a bug in a rug' and want to stay living there.

There are many potential ways to restore the delicate balance in the intestine. The central approach is to always supply the good gut bacteria with what they need. The largest groups of good bacteria in the intestine are the bifidobacteria and the lactobacilli. For this reason, these two bacteria species are very common in probiotic products for building up the intestinal flora.

The most reasonably priced and most natural way to consume gut bacteria is in **sauerkraut or pickled vegetables**. You can either make them yourself or buy them ready made at the store. Sauerkraut is finely cut raw cabbage that has been fermented by certain lactic acid bacteria.

However, caution is advised when buying it in the store, because sauerkraut either in a can or in a jar is preserved to make it last for a long time. This preservation process means that it no longer contains any living bacteria. But in order to build up the intestinal flora, we need exactly these living bacteria. Therefore, a measurement of good sauerkraut or pickled vegetables is that it should be as fresh as possible and it´s shelf life is no longer than two or three weeks. Only then it will have a good impact on the intestinal flora.

Another option to pep up the intestinal flora is by consuming **probiotic products**. These are products available in capsule, powder or liquid form that contain several types of gut bacteria. The disadvantage in comparison to sauerkraut or any pickled vegetable is of course the price. However, these products also have a big advantage: They usually contain many different species of bacteria. The reason why probiotics should contain as many different bacterial species as possible, is that there are not only two or three different species of bacteria in our intestine, but several thousand.

A good probiotic product is not only distinguished by the number of different bacterial strains; the total number of the bacteria also plays a role. This is because it makes a huge difference, whether you are consuming one thousand, one million or even one billion bacteria with a single capsule.

Another important aspect of choosing a probiotic is that it should contain as few additives as possible. This is an important point for a damaged intestine. Unfortunately, most products contain additives, which are of questionable value even for a healthy person. Especially someone with a damaged gut should absolutely avoid any unnecessary additives, because they can get into the blood much faster due to the permeability of the intestine.

There is something else very important when you are consuming probiotic products, but it is also concerning sauerkraut and pickled vegetables – it is the matter of **histamine**. All of these products can lead to digestive problems when you are histamine intolerant. If you are not sure, then you should check first if you have a histamine intolerance. Anyone who is histamine intolerant should therefore avoid sauerkraut, pickled vegetables and only select those probiotics that are specifically made for histamine intolerance.

Since histamine plays a very important role for many people with an irritable bowel nowadays, we will take a closer look at histamine in the following.

Info-Box 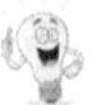

- ✓ Things that damage the intestinal flora are antibiotics, preservatives, poor nutrition (especially too much sugar and white flour), stress and excessive hygiene
- ✓ The pH value in the intestine should be in the range between 5.8 and 6.5, so that the "good" bacteria feel really well
- ✓ It is very useful to take a laboratory test for intruders (viruses, bacteria, worms or fungi)
- ✓ Good things for pepping up the intestinal flora include probiotic products, sauerkraut or pickled vegetables

3.4 Histamine: Tiny hormones with a lot of power

Now we have seen that even very tiny gut bacteria can have a very big impact. It is hard to imagine that even such miniscule components in the body can have such grave consequences on our health. However, gut bacteria are not the only tiny things that can have a big impact: Histamine is also invisible to the naked eye and can nevertheless have unforeseen consequences.

The term "histamine intolerance" has gotten a real hype lately. Until a few years ago, histamine intolerance was something completely unknown and was not regarded as anything associated with digestive problems. Nevertheless, because the growing number of people with a diagnosed histamine intolerance, the more science and laboratories are concerned with researching about histamine intolerance.

For most intolerances, it is quite clear which foods should be avoided. For lactose intolerance (= milk sugar) it is mostly dairy products; for gluten intolerance you should avoid grain products. But which foods contain histamine? This question is not that easy to answer.

To explain this complexity a little more, we take a freshwater fish like salmon for an example. Right after the fish is caught, it contains practically no histamine. However, fish spoils quickly and this degradation process can produce a lot of histamine within a short amount of time. Besides, it also depends on the type of fish: Freshwater fish contain almost no histamine, while canned fishes or seafood contain a large amount of histamine. And the processing method is also crucial: If the fish has been smoked, it contains significantly more histamine than if it is not smoked.

Thus, the histamine problem is not such an easy one and taking a closer look at histamine is worth its while, because many people with an intolerance feel much better once they have realized what products are rich in histamine and once they have eliminated them.

Foods that are produced by fermentation usually contain a lot of histamine. Some examples are cheese, sausage, sauerkraut, yeast extract, wine and beer. Slowly cured sausages and ripened cheeses in particular contain significantly more histamine than young, less-aged products. Due to the longer ripening process, the microorganisms are able to remain active over a longer period of time and thus more protein is converted into histamine. Besides these foods, there are a lot more that contain large quantities of histamine. One major rule of thumb when it comes to histamine is: **The fresher, the better**!

But why is histamine in particular so closely associated with IBS? To answer this question, we have to look a little deeper into the natural processes in the body. In order to react to external influences or intruders, the body can set off an inflammation, which warms up the tissue in the affected area and makes more blood flow there. This means that more constructive substances arrive and waste materials are removed faster. This leads to real motion within the affected area in order to heal it or to fight invaders.

However, for an inflammation to arise at all, the body has to send certain signal substances to this place. These substances ensure that inflammation can be initiated or that an existing inflammation will be sustained. There are many different types of these signal substances and they are generally called "inflammatory mediators." These inflammatory mediators include prostaglandins, leukotrienes and ... you guessed it – histamine. This means, that the body stores histamine and can release it on its own when it needs histamine, so that an inflammation can develop or a certain area remains inflamed.

When you eat a food that contains a lot of histamine and you can´t break down this histamine sufficiently due to your histamine intolerance, then the result is an excess of histamine in your body. This excess can lead to inflammation in the intestine, since histamine is an inflammatory mediator. This intestinal inflammation then expands the distance between the intestinal cells and digestive disorders arise. Based on these correlations, we can see that IBS and histamine can be very closely associated with each other.

Creating an inflammation is just one characteristics of histamine. It can also control gastric acid, the sleep-wake rhythm, appetite, heart rate and many more functions.

So, the fundamental problem with histamine intolerance is that the body is unable to sufficiently break down the histamine that is either released within the body or is contained in food. What then prevails is an imbalance between the formation and breakdown of histamine.

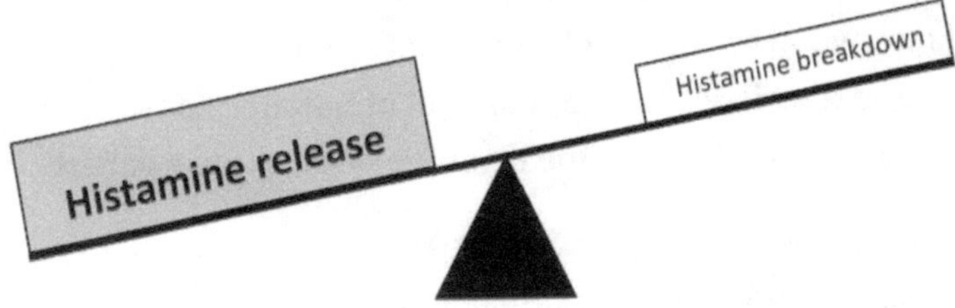

While healthy people will have no problem with histamine-rich foods, for people with histamine intolerance these foods can put their entire wellbeing out of balance.

Histamine intolerance can be triggered in three different ways:

1) By eating foods that contain a lot of histamine themselves;
2) By eating foods or taking medicines that in fact contain almost no histamine themselves, but release the histamine stored in the body. They are called histamine liberators;
3) By consuming certain active ingredients such as those in energy drinks or alcohol, that prevent the breakdown of histamine in the body by blocking the DAO enzyme.

How do you measure histamine intolerance?

If you are currently struggling with IBS, it is very important to know whether you are histamine intolerant or not. If you still keep eating foods that contain a lot of histamine despite your histamine intolerance, the digestive disorders will persist.

Just like with other intolerances, the most reliable and at the same time the least expensive method to test for histamine intolerance is the **elimination diet**. To do this, you should avoid all foods that contain a lot of histamine for about one to two weeks. If your symptoms improve significantly during this time, it is quite likely that you are histamine intolerant.

While on the elimination diet, it is a good idea to keep a diary on your nutrition and symptoms. This gives you a good overview of which foods you have eaten throughout the day and whether they have caused any symptoms. This also makes it easier to identify associations between what you eat and any digestive problems over a longer period of time. After eating a specific food or meal, it can sometimes take 24 to 48 hours before you will notice any symptoms, which makes it very difficult to figure out which foods are causing problems. Besides this, a therapist or nutritionist can look at your diary and check on whether you have in fact accidentally eaten something wrong.

As already mentioned, it is not that easy to determine what foods are rich in histamine. A list of all histamine-rich foods here would definitely go beyond the scope of IBS discussion. However, there are detailed tables on the Internet with hundreds of foods and their histamine content. Another practical way is to use a histamine app on your smartphone. It helps you identify histamine-rich foods on the go and when you need it most, for example when you are grocery shopping or at a restaurant.

As a short introduction into the topic of histamine foods, I would like to just note some typical "histamine bombs":

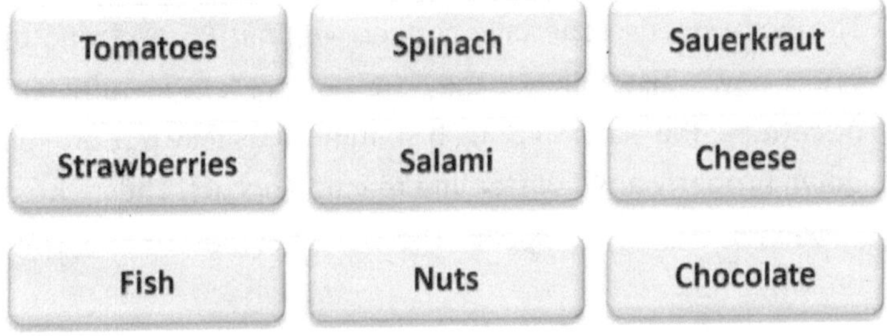

In addition to the elimination diet, it is also possible to test for histamine intolerance by means of laboratory values. To do this, the **DAO values in the blood** should be checked. DAO (Di-amine Oxidase) is an enzyme in the body that takes care of breaking down histamine.

If there is too little DAO present, the histamine is not broken down sufficiently. Since the DAO value can fluctuate considerably during the day, it should be measured at least twice. If multiple measurements are taken, the daily fluctuations no longer carry so much weight and the significance of the measurement is therefore definitely more reliable.

Besides the DAO value, it is also possible to get a hint about a histamine intolerance by identifying the **copper, vitamin B6 and zinc** values in whole blood. Just be sure to always have your vitamin and mineral levels measured in whole blood instead in serum. Some laboratories also call this method "intracellular," because it looks inside your cells.

The body needs especially copper, vitamin B6 and zinc to break down histamine. If they are not present in sufficient quantities, the accumulating histamine is usually not broken down properly and a histamine reaction occurs. These three nutrients are, so to speak, the best buddies of the DAO enzyme.

A third method to determine histamine intolerance is to measure the **methylhistamine** in 24-hour urine. A single measurement of histamine in urine would not be meaningful, since the value fluctuates a lot over the day, depending on what you ate. However, if you look at the average over 24 hours, the measurement becomes significantly more reliable. But this method of measuring methylhistamine in 24-hour urine is not so common and I would rather start with an elimination diet as well as checking the DAO value in the blood.

Besides measuring the DAO level, it is also meaningful to measure the histamine level in the blood. In most laboratories, this is called "**total histamine level**" or "histamine in plasma." But why is it important to measure the total histamine level? It could be that your DAO level is fine and you can break down histamine without any problems, but for some reason your body releases excessive amounts of histamine. This can be the case if you have a type I allergy or you are taking certain medications.

So, it could be the case, that you have a good DAO value and your process to breakdown histamine is working perfectly well, but the amount of histamine in your body is just way too high. Therefore, the laboratory value of "total histamine level" will give you a good indication of that. If your histamine levels are far above normal, then you only need to figure out what causes this excessive release of histamine in your body.

However, this value alone is very unreliable, because the histamine level in the blood depends very much on what you have just eaten beforehand. If you had tuna and tomato the night before, it could be that the test will find a very high level of histamine in the blood. If you had only eaten potatoes or rice the evening before, then the histamine level in the blood would likely be significantly low. Therefore, you have to eat a low-histamine diet one or two days prior to testing the total histamine value, and you should repeat that test in order to get a good, reliable result.

In conclusion, there are two very reliable ways of testing for histamine intolerance: One is the elimination diet and the other one is a laboratory test for DAO as well as the "total histamine level" in the blood.

What can you do about histamine intolerance?

If it turns out from the tests that you are histamine intolerant, then this might sound depressing at the first moment. However, this isn't just bad news, because now you have a clear indication about the cause of your digestive problems.

It is very important to point out again that you shouldn´t just suppress the histamine symptoms or live on a histamine-free diet for the rest of your life. We have to get one level deeper to the root cause in order to cure the disease over the long term.

The causes of histamine intolerance are, for the most part, similar to the causes of digestive problems in general. If you remedy the cause of your histamine intolerance, then in most cases this eliminates the cause of the digestive disorders at the same time. There aren't an infinite number of causes for IBS, food intolerance, leaky gut or histamine intolerance. It is mostly the usual suspects. Digestive problems can in fact take a different form in every person. Some have diarrhea, abdominal pain or bloating, others have flatulence, itchy skin and so on, but their underlying causes are often the same:

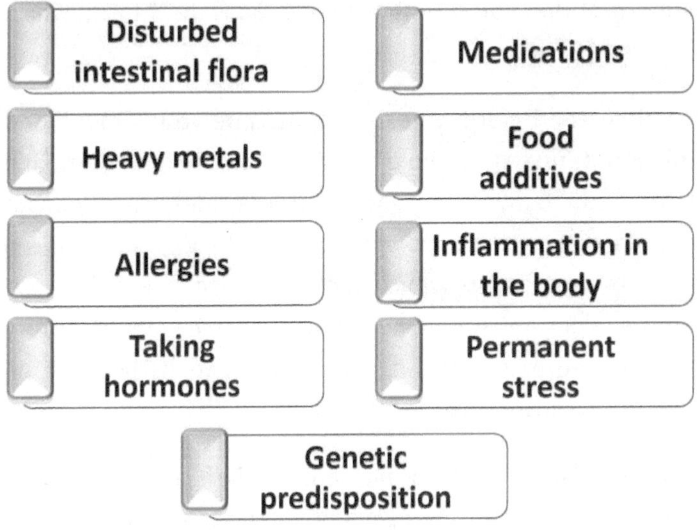

After you get the diagnosis of histamine intolerance, the first and most important step is to **adapt your diet**. This is very important and this is the only way that the irritated intestine can calm down.

As already mentioned, there is an enzyme that does a lot of histamine-related work and it takes care of breaking down histamine – this is the DAO enzyme. For DAO to work well, it needs its friends to help it in this work: **Copper, zinc, vitamin C and activated vitamin B6 (P-5-P)**. If these substances are lacking, the body cannot break down the histamine sufficiently – the result is histamine intolerance. However, a deficiency can be easily remedied by food supplements. When you supplement your vitamin B6, it is important that you take the already "activated" form, which is called *"P-5-P."*

As discussed before, you should measure your vitamin and mineral status in the whole blood first, before taking any kind of food supplement. For example, if your zinc level is fine, but you start taking zinc supplements over a longer time, this will lead to an overdose which can cause negative effects. So before taking any supplement, you need to have a laboratory test to figure out first if you really need it, because an overdose is just as bad as a deficiency.

However, if you get a nutrient analysis done, I would recommend **measuring as many nutrients and vitamins as possible**. This gives you a complete overview and you won't miss anything. I would recommend testing for:

Chromium	**Vitamin A**
Manganese	**Vitamin C**
Sodium	**Vitamin E**
Calium	**Vitamin D (25 OH)**
Magnesium	**Vitamin K**
Calcium	**Vitamin B1**
Copper	**Vitamin B2**
Iron	**Vitamin B3**
Zinc	**Vitamin B6**
Selenium	**Vitamin B12**
Biotin	**Coenzym Q10**
Folic acid	

Especially vitamin D and vitamin B12 are very important in context of histamine intolerance and for overall health as well.

If you struggle with histamine intolerance and the symptoms get really bad, there are certain emergency medications to suppress these symptoms. The medications for that are called "**antihistamines**" and they bind themselves to a histamine receptor in the body. The histamine is then still released, but it can no longer settle anywhere because the antihistamine medications have already occupied the histamine receptor. This lessens the severity of symptoms such as redness or sneezing, but the histamine is still released anyway.

That's why you should only take these medications in an emergency and not over a longer time. When taking antihistamines, you won´t notice most symptoms anymore and it feels like you are healed. But what really happens in the background is that only the symptoms are blocked and there is still too much histamine released in your body.

Besides this, there are medications which help break down the released histamine. They contain artificial DAO enzymes which help to break down histamine in the intestine before it gets into the blood. This is already better than taking an antihistamine, but it doesn't change the histamine intolerance in any way. It may even be the case that the body might get used to taking artificial DAO enzymes and as a result it produces even less DAO itself.

However, these artificial DAO products are not helpful with all kind of foods. There are certain foods, drinks or medications that do not contain any histamine themselves, but instead trigger a histamine reaction by releasing the histamine stored in the body. These foods are called "*histamine liberators*." In such cases, DAO medications are of no help.

Antihistamines as well as DAO products should therefore only be considered as a stopgap solution, because they can have side effects and don't solve any of the existing problems – they only suppress the symptoms.

However, it is possible to improve digestive problems a little bit in a natural way: Through regular **exercise**. At the same time, exercise stimulates the metabolic processes in the entire body and significantly improves digestive performance. The best evidence that exercise has a positive effect on digestion is the ravenous appetite you get after strenuous physical activity. If you are histamine intolerant, however, you should be careful about very exhausting kinds of sports because this releases additional histamine in the body.

To find a happy medium, you only have to pay attention to the symptoms during or after exercise. If you get the typical histamine symptoms, then it was too much and you are doing yourself more harm than the exercise did your health any good. Moderate exercise, on the other hand, is very beneficial for digestion – especially on a regular basis and not only during the Christmas holidays!

Info-Box 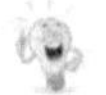

- ✓ It is important to identify the cause of histamine intolerance
- ✓ You can find out if you are histamine intolerant by
    - An elimination diet (eliminate histamine-rich foods)
    - Check the DAO value and total histamine level in the blood (measure at least twice)
    - Copper, vitamin B6 and zinc levels (in whole blood)
- ✓ Certain vitamins and minerals are very important for breaking down histamine. They should be checked and supplemented if too low: Copper, zinc, vitamin C and activated vitamin B6 (P-5-P)
- ✓ Gentle exercise is beneficial and good for the digestion; excessive sports on the other hand cause the release of additional histamine

3.5 A thorough spring cleaning: Free your body of harmful heavy metals

When talking about heavy metals in the body, you most likely just think about miners who constantly come into contact with metals and ores in the mine. In fact, heavy metals have become so common in our everyday lives that nowadays anyone can be affected. Unfortunately, there are no concrete indications or symptoms which clearly point to heavy metal poisoning.

The tricky thing about heavy metals is that they accumulate in the body very slowly and over time. Additionally, the body has very few options for ridding itself of heavy metals. Normally, our body is an absolute marvel and it has adapted to a whole lot of environmental conditions over the long history of mankind. Human beings can survive in space; they can survive in the Arctic at extremely low temperatures, as well as in the desert in severe heat. From generation to generation, the human body has been able to adapt better and better to certain environmental conditions.

On the other hand, it has not been able to get used to heavy metals so far. This is mainly because heavy metals were buried beneath the earth for many millennia. It is only in the past few decades that heavy metals have been used in large quantities by industry and have thus been rapidly distributed.

When you have accumulated too many heavy metals in your body, it usually isn't possible to determine afterwards just exactly what was the source of that heavy metal toxicity. Often it is simply a result of everyday contact with these metals. Since you can't see heavy metals, you can't smell and you can't taste them, you often don't even notice their existence.

In our environment, there are heavy metals lurking all over the place: In fish from the oceans, in aluminum saucepans, vaccinations, amalgam fillings, you can find them in drinking water or any kind of food. Since heavy metals are so widespread nowadays, in principle almost everyone is affected by heavy metal toxicity. The question is therefore not whether you have heavy metals in your body. It is much more important what amounts of these metals are lying dormant in your body and whether the quantity is already large enough so that it makes you sick.

The problem is that heavy metals work on a very fundamental, deep level and they block the normal function of our cells. We have cells throughout our entire body and that is why the symptoms of heavy metal toxicity can appear so totally different.

You can think of heavy metal toxicity like a water tap. In most taps, there is a fine strainer on the end. If more and more deposits build up in this strainer over time, the water flows much more slowly. The larger the deposits in the strainer, the less water can flow through it.

The heavy metals act the same way in your cells. Once they have entered the cell, they disrupt the immune cells and induce them to react incorrectly. The best example of such faulty reactions are autoimmune diseases, in which the immune defense is directed against the body's own tissue. Furthermore, heavy metals can damage the nerves within a cell or they block receptors that are actually reserved for messenger substances and hormones. Thus, heavy metals can do immense damage to the body.

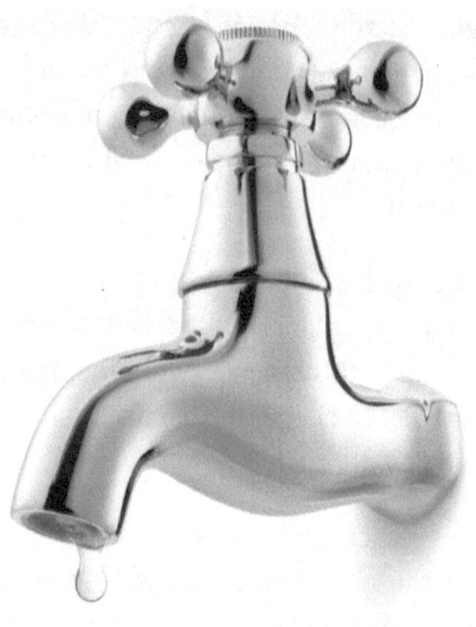

From my experience, I would therefore classify heavy metals high up among the causes of IBS. There are meanwhile countless reports of patients who have been able to make enormous progress in healing their digestive problems by heavy metal detoxification.

How can you measure heavy metal toxicity?
A fairly large market comprising various suppliers of tests for heavy metals has developed in the meantime. However, many of these tests provide completely false results. An example of false testing is to take a heavy metal measurement from the blood or from hair. A measurement from a hair sample only tells you how much heavy metal is stored in your hair. In principle, the body can store heavy

metals anywhere and since you get your hair cut, this measurement can only provide information about the last few weeks or months.

The case is similar when taking a measurement from blood. The body does not store the metals in the blood and constantly carry them all around the body; instead, it prefers to store them in tissue. Since heavy metals are stored somewhere in the tissues, you will not get anywhere by taking a measurement from blood.

There are all sorts of very adventurous methods for measuring a heavy metal toxicity: From vibration machines to lighting devices, anything and everything is available nowadays. Yet you don't have to be satisfied with such bad testing procedures, because there is a very reliable and scientific method out there: The **provocative chelation test.** It provides a method which environmental physicians currently regard as the most reliable method of heavy metal testing and therapy as well [5]. As a patient, you don't have to do very much. You only have to wait until the infusion with DMSO and EDTA has passed through you. In most cases, this takes about 1.5 to 2 hours. After that, a urine sample is taken and sent to a laboratory. This provocative chelation test for heavy metals can be performed by a specialist doctor or a natural practitioner.

To get a better idea of how chelates work, you can think of a bowl filled with cotton balls and paper clips. If you now pass a magnet through the bowl, it only attracts the paper clips but the cotton balls remain in the bowl. In the body, the chelates work exactly the same: They circulate through your whole body and attract metals. In this way, they act like a magnet.

The collected heavy metals are then excreted in the urine and the results can be analyzed in the laboratory. If this method is used, it doesn't matter at all where exactly the body has stored the heavy metals. The chelates get into every corner of the body via the circulating blood and can then bind the heavy metals.

What can you do if you have too many heavy metals in your body?

To measure a heavy metal toxicity, the urine is collected after the chelation infusion and is sent to a laboratory. This is how you measure the level of the heavy metal toxicity in your body. If one or even more heavy metal values are notably high, then treatment follows. The treatment works pretty much by using the same process and you likewise get chelation infusions. The only difference is that your urine is not sent to the laboratory afterwards.

Before deciding on a chelation treatment, it is absolutely essential to check whether your kidneys are functioning properly. Kidney function is measured by checking the "**cystantin C**" level and this can be done by your general practitioner. Since heavy metals are excreted in the urine, a good kidney function here is very important.

However, it takes a little patience to remove the heavy metals. Most people have had a certain amount of heavy metals deposited over time in their body and the chelates can only absorb a certain quantity of metals at a time. This is similar to our example of the magnet which is pulled through the bowl and attracts the metallic paper clips.

When the magnet becomes completely covered at some point, no more paper clips will cling to it. Then you need a new magnet. Likewise, the chelates absorb metals in the body until they are saturated and that is the reason why you cannot remove all heavy metals with a single chelation treatment.

Furthermore, it is important that a replacement infusion containing **minerals** is administered directly after each chelate treatment. The reason behind the replacement infusion right after the chelate therapy is that the chelates also remove some beneficial minerals. After the chelate treatment, you don´t want to end up with a major lack of good minerals and that´s why refilling your body with them afterwards is so important.

In addition to chelation treatment, it is also possible to remove heavy metals by using herbs. Wild garlic, coriander and chlorella algae work well for this. However, this treatment has two decisive disadvantages compared to the chelation treatment. The herbs first have to pass through the entire gastrointestinal tract and therefore a certain portion of them is already lost in the intestine. Also, the heavy metal binding is mainly restricted to the intestine. Therefore, detoxification from heavy metals by using herbs can sometimes take a very long time.

IBS patients already have an intestine that is already very upset and sensitive. Therefore, it would not be advisable for someone with digestive problems to try a herbal cure through their intestine. In contrast, chelates are administered by infusion. This means that they are infused directly into the blood, so they can collect metals anywhere in the body and do not irritate the intestine.

The second major disadvantage particularly of chlorella algae is that it can be heavily contaminated with heavy metals even before you take it. These algae are cultivated in water. Due to its strong capacity to attract heavy metals, the chlorella algae may become saturated with heavy metals when it is grown in contaminated water. This way, you are adding additional heavy metals to your body through the chlorella algae and you achieve exactly the opposite of what you want.

Heavy metal detoxification is very important to get rid of existing metals and many people with IBS have already benefited enormously from this procedure. However, the detoxification process is just as important as prevention in order to accumulate as few heavy metals as possible. Nowadays, it isn't possible to avoid contact with heavy metals completely, but you can significantly minimize the risk.

A pretty large amount of heavy metals can come from water in particular. To avoid this, I am using a water filter with activated carbon and ion exchanger. This filters out more than 99 percent of lime, heavy metals and drug residues.

Concerning water filters in general, it is important that the water is only filtered by gravity and not with any additional pressure, since this will not alter the natural properties of the water structure. Besides this, the filters need to be replaceable and should be changed at certain intervals. A replaceable filter is not part of every filter system, but it really helps reducing the risk of germs and bacteria, which can accumulate in the filter very quickly over time.

Info-Box

- ✓ The best method to test for heavy metal toxicity is the provocative chelation test
- ✓ Before using chelates to remove heavy metals, the kidney function has to be checked first by *"cystantin C"* value
- ✓ When the laboratory test shows, that the heavy metal load in the body is too high, then the best way to remove them is by a chelate infusion
- ✓ On the long run, it is important to avoid further heavy metal toxification, especially from foods and water

3.6 HPU – When your metabolism doesn't run smoothly

Oh, boy ... another technical term ... HPU! Fortunately, the abbreviation "HPU" has become generally accepted instead of its long form *"**h**emo**p**yrrollactam**u**ria."* HPU is a metabolic disorder and if it is left untreated, it can lead to constant digestive problems. Although there are many different metabolic disorders such as diabetes, hyperthyroidism or gout, HPU is linked particularly closely to the development of digestive problems.

A metabolic disorder – that sounds pretty dramatic at first – but in fact, HPU is not that severe. The test for HPU doesn´t hurt at all and once it is identified, there are several things you can do about it. The most decisive factor about HPU is identifying it in the first place. HPU disease is usually inherited, but it can also develop over the course of life and women are affected 10 times more often than men are.

Let´s take a closer look at HPU disease. When we breathe in, oxygen enters our lungs. This oxygen must then be distributed all over the body through the blood stream and that is done by the red blood cells. More precisely, the oxygen binds to hemoglobin. This hemoglobin is like a pack donkey and transports oxygen everywhere in the body. As the name already suggests, hemoglobin consists of heme (an iron complex) and globin (a protein compound). The body can produce both heme and globin itself.

In case of HPU disease, the production of this heme becomes disrupted. As a result of this disorder, a certain amount of "false" heme is formed and the body naturally wants to get rid of this "false" heme. In order to do this, it has to bind this false heme to vitamin B6, zinc and sometimes also to manganese so that it can excrete it in the urine.

People with HPU metabolic disorder form a certain portion of this "false" heme every day. This means that the body has to take some of the vital substance's vitamin B6, zinc and manganese every day in order to just dispose the "false" heme.

Thus, over time the body loses more and more vital substances that are actually required for other processes as well. In addition to the "false" heme, the body is also simultaneously encumbered with other contaminants from the environment. Due to HPU, it is much more difficult to get rid of these other contaminants, since the body has already used the necessary nutrients to dispose of the "false" heme. That means, HPU creates two problem areas at the same time: A lack of nutrients (vitamin B6, zinc, manganese) as well as limited detoxification performance.

How to measure HPU?

HPU can be measured easily by a **24-hour urine test**. To do this, you simply collect the urine over 24 hours and then send a small sample of it to the laboratory[1]. The excretion of HPU complexes can vary widely over the day, but the 24-hour test won't be affected by this. By collecting the urine over 24 hours, these fluctuations during the day will be effectively balanced out and you get a reliable test result.

Sometimes the so-called KPU test is used to measure HPU disease. The KPU test measures the kryptopyrroluria complexes. Even they might sound very similar, the KPU test is different from HPU test and can be distorted by certain foods, medications or stress and might therefore bring out a false-positive result. The HPU test, on the other hand, measures a very special chemical compound that only arises when "false" heme is formed, independent of what you ate before. Unfortunately, KPU testing is still quite often equated with the HPU test. This is maybe because they both sound alike, but the HPU test is the more reliable of the two.

It should be noted that no food supplements, such as B-Vitamins or zinc, should be taken for about two weeks before the HPU test, because they can falsify the test result.

---

[1]A laboratory that carries out the HPU test is the KEAC laboratory (https://www.keac.nl).

What can you do about HPU?

If the test has shown that HPU metabolic disorder is present, then you have to replenish your emptied deposits of nutrients. These include in particular vitamin B6, zinc and manganese. As a result, the body emerges from its exhausting state of deficiency. Since it is so important, I must again note at this point: When taking vitamin B6, you should make sure that you are always taking the **activated Vitamin B6 (P-5-P)**.

Since people who have HPU usually lack several nutrients, it is advisable to take a supplement that contains all the B vitamins ("vitamin B complex") for a certain length of time.

At first glance, taking food supplements does not appear to be a spectacular treatment concept for HPU. But in case of HPU metabolic disorder, the lack of certain nutrients is exactly the crux of the matter as to why certain processes have been thrown out of kilter. It would be ideal, of course, to treat the original cause of the HPU. However, since it is often genetically determined, there is not much that can be changed about the actual cause.

But there is even more that can be done than just taking food supplements. As mentioned above, the detoxification performance is limited with HPU. Therefore, someone with HPU should be particularly careful about what they eat. Their food should be as natural as possible and above all without any sprayed toxins. Heavy metals in particular have an even greater impact on anyone who has HPU.

In relation to heavy metals, you should also be careful about getting vaccinations because they contain aluminum. The shot takes the aluminum directly into the blood and the body has no way of protecting itself. Besides this, taking certain medications or electro smog can affect people with HPU more than a healthy person due to the limited detoxification performance.

3.7 The leaky gut syndrome

If you take a closer look at the intestine, then it becomes apparent that it has to perform at full capacity every day. After we enjoyed a nice meal, the food passes through various digestive stations: The mouth, the stomach, the gall bladder, the pancreas and, last but not least, the intestine. No matter what your dinner looked like before, now it's just a food mush. One task of the intestine is to release enzymes that break down sugars, such as lactose (=milk sugar) or fructose (=fruit sugar). Only when all the components of the food are broken down into their smallest parts, can they be transferred into the blood.

At this point, the processes in the gut are getting really exciting. There are not only vital nutrients in our food, but some unpleasant fellows have also been smuggled in: Viruses, bacteria, pathogens, as well as chemical contaminants from the environment. Here, the intestine acts like a bouncer. It has to watch out very carefully about what is allowed to enter your bloodstream and what is not.

To guard against intruders, there are three protective systems in the intestine. The first protection system is the **mucous membrane**. This extends for many meters, from the mouth to the anus. The bacteria that live on this mucous membrane are the second protective barrier. In the intestine, these are the **gut bacteria**, which have become pretty famous during recent years. The gut bacteria have many tasks to fulfill and one of these tasks is to fight against unwanted intruders and kill them off. If an intruder passes these first two systems, mucous membrane and gut bacteria, it still has to fight with the third protective device – and this is the **intestines' own immune system**. As you can see, the body has thus developed a very sophisticated system over tens of thousands of years to ward off foreign substances.

The intestine's most important task is to absorb nutrients and pass them into the blood. However, if the cells in the intestine were simply strung closely together, we would not be able to absorb nutrients from our food. For this reason, there is a kind of intermediate space with a filter between each two cells in the intestinal mucosa. These intermediate spaces are called **tight junctions**. The tight junctions work in a way similar to a tea filter made of paper: Some substances can pass through, while others by contrast are held back.

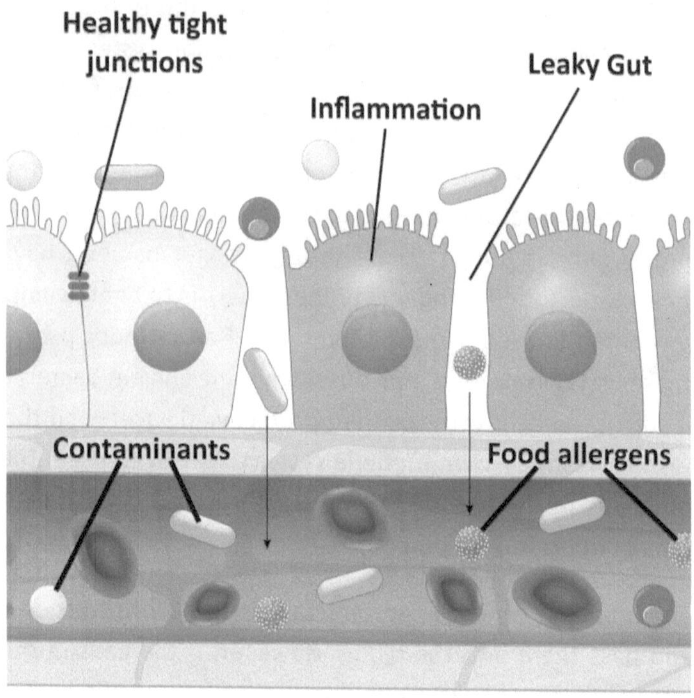

Figure 1: The tight junctions in a healthy gut (left side) and in a leaking gut (right side).

However, there are situations in which such a reaction is very useful for the body. In an extreme situation, the body needs nutrients very quickly. To achieve this, the intestine becomes more permeable, more nutrients can be quickly absorbed into the blood and you are best prepared to take flight over a long distance.

It is not much of a problem when the intestine becomes permeable for just a short time. This is a completely normal process. The dilemma only begins when this condition persists, because then a large number of disease-causing substances can enter the bloodstream unnoticed.

When a leaky gut persists, in many cases the intestinal mucosa becomes inflamed. This is the body's emergency program for dealing with intruders. Therefore, in most cases the intestine is not only permeable, but also inflamed at the same time. Permeability and inflammation thus are usually very closely associated. As long as the intestine remains permeable, the inflammation persists just as long.

You can already recognize the characteristics of an inflammation from the original root word. Inflammation means that something in the body is literally "in flames." Like a fire, an inflammation is characterized by redness and heat. This reaction is an indication that the body is putting up a fight against something.

When you are suffering from a leaky gut syndrome, you are definitely not alone out there. But it is not possible to say exactly how many people there are who have a leaky gut. This is because in conventional medical practice, patients with unexplained abdominal pain and digestive problems are usually not examined to check for a leaky gut and medical statistics do not include any group for leaky gut. Therefore, these patients fall somewhere in the "irritable bowel group." Alone in Germany, there are between 8 million to 9 million irritable bowel patients [1]. Eight million people affected by irritable bowel syndrome comprise a frighteningly high number – that's about 10% of the population and therefore it is definitely not a rare disease.

How to measure leaky gut syndrome?

The body needs to be able to open and close the tight junctions, and this happens by the means of a protein called **zonulin**. The term zonulin is very important for people who would like to know if they have a leaky gut, because the zonulin value makes it possible to clearly determine whether someone is suffering from leaky gut syndrome or not.

If there is too much zonulin in the intestine, then the tight junctions constantly get the signal to open up the space between two cells. The term "leaky gut" indicates already the core of the problem: The intestine is "permeable" or "holey," and therefore something is leaking that normally should be leak-proof.

What can you do about leaky gut syndrome?

A leaky gut is not the actual cause for digestive disorders and there has to be another reason that causes the leaky gut.

When you check the result of your stool sample and you recognize that your zonulin level is elevated, you know then that you are suffering from a leaky gut. However, at this point you shouldn´t stop the investigations. The next step is to find out what causes the body to end up with this leaky gut. It is something like a chain or an interconnection: A certain cause makes the intestine permeable and as a result, this causes IBS.

Since a leaky gut very often comes with inflammation, a lot of measures against intestinal inflammation from *Chapter 3.1 Good remedies against inflammation* can help, so that at least the inflammation calms down. It is an important aspect to reduce the inflammation, because it makes the intestine permeable.

Bringing down the inflammation can already help you to feel much better or to be able to eat some more foods that you could not handle before. However, the main goal is to find the root cause behind that leaky gut. In most cases, the main reasons for a leaky gut are the same as for IBS in general: Your gut bacteria can be out of balance, your pancreas is weakened, you have histamine intolerance and many more. Therefore, the main focus should not be on the leaky gut itself, but rather on healing the underlying cause behind the leaky gut.

3.8 Legal doping for the pancreas

Although IBS affects the intestine, the cause for it can lie somewhere totally different. We have already seen this with heavy metals and it is a similar situation for the pancreas. Here too, inadequate functioning can affect the intestine and since everything in the body is interrelated, you often have to think outside the box to figure out the cause of certain diseases.

Just like the intestine, the pancreas is also a digestive organ and it is part of the digestive chain. It´s main task is to release enzymes to break down proteins, carbohydrates and fats. If the pancreas is working well, the components of your food are broken down very finely.

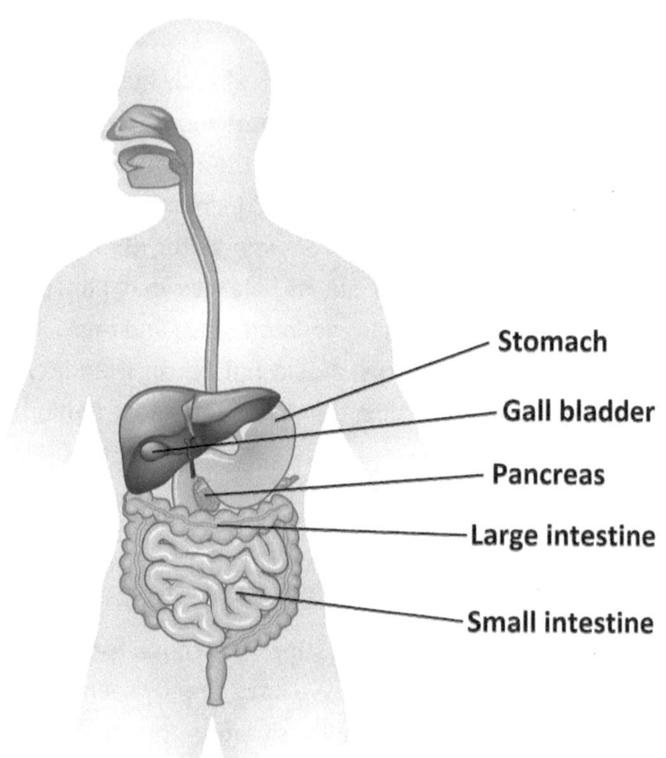

However, if the pancreas is weakened and releases too little enzymes, the food is in a form that is much too coarse when it arrives in the intestine. As a result, the intestine is completely overwhelmed.

The poorly digested food then remains in the intestine for a long time and fermentation processes start. Over the long run, this changes the pH in the intestine and above all, it changes the composition of the intestinal flora to the worse. These fermentation processes make their presence felt primarily as flatulence or abdominal pain. The "bad" bacteria feel very comfortable in this fermenting chaos and spread rapidly. In contrast, the "good" gut bacteria find the whole thing not much to their taste and they cannot spread well in this environment. And as we have already seen earlier, an excess of "bad" bacteria in the gut can lead to digestive disorders.

Before you start thinking that there is something really wrong with your pancreas: We're just talking about a weakness of the pancreas, not about an inflammation. An inflammation often makes its presence felt in the form of stinging pain in the abdominal area. In contrast, you will usually be completely unaware of weakness of the pancreas. Now, let's take a closer look at how to figure out if your pancreas is weakened.

You can imagine the function of the pancreas by thinking of the dishwashing liquid you use when cleaning the dishes. If you have a very large sink and only add a single drop of detergent, it is really hard to get rid of the dirt on your dishes.

Most things keep sticking on and washing the dishes becomes a tedious ordeal. On the other hand, if you add a hefty amount of detergent, you will have no problem in cleaning the remains of food from the dishes and little effort is required.

Things are very similar concerning the pancreas. If it releases only a very small amount of its secretions, then it becomes impossible to break down the components of food. They get into the intestine in very coarse form and ultimately, it is the intestine that has to suffer the consequences of a weakened pancreas. Therefore, taking a closer look at the pancreas is definitely worthwhile when searching for the cause of digestive problems.

The following example also makes it very clear just how closely all the processes in the body are interconnected: If someone suffers from heartburn, most doctors prescribe a stomach acid blocker (also called proton pump inhibitor). This will greatly reduce the production of stomach acid or even stop it completely.

However, this intervention will have consequences in an unexpected direction. Due to the stomach acid blocker, there is hardly any stomach acid available and food will of course not be broken down sufficiently in the stomach. This means that this digestive step in the stomach is skipped and this is only the beginning in terms of the side effects of a stomach acid blocker.

The pancreas doesn't just simply release enzymes indiscriminately all day long. It waits for a signal that tells it when food is on the way and when it really makes sense to release the enzymes. The pancreas gets this signal from the acidic gastric juices, particularly by the very low pH value of the stomach acid.

If there are no gastric juices due to the stomach acid blocker, then the pancreas doesn't receive a signal that it should release its secretions. Thus, taking a stomach acid blocker puts the stomach as well as the pancreas out of commission at the same time. The intestine then takes over the entire digestive process all by itself.

Because of these complex relationships in the body, we should never consider IBS separately from other processes. A malfunction or lack in one part of the body can have serious consequences in a completely different place.

How do you measure whether the pancreas is weakened?

Measuring how well the pancreas works is not difficult at all. Here, our most powerful weapon comes into play once again: The stool sample. In addition to many other values related to the intestine, the stool sample can also be used at the same time to determine the performance of the pancreas. This is done by measuring the **pancreatic elastase** value.

For pancreatic elastase, however, we should be careful with using just one single value. This measurement can really fluctuate a lot and therefore it is advisable to check it at least two or three times.

What can you do about a weak pancreas?

Over the centuries, **bitter substances** have already proven their worth to really get the upper digestive organs going. They really boost the digestive capacity of the stomach, gall bladder and pancreas.

Now, many men will probably jump up happily and say: "*Beer has a lot of bitter substances.... Let´s have three or four to boost my digestion.*" At first glance, this sounds like a good idea, but in turn, the alcohol in beer isn't beneficial for the pancreas at all. Too much alcohol in particular is one major reason for a weakened pancreas. Therefore, **bitter digestive herbs** are a much better choice.

To really get the weakened pancreas going again, **pancreatic enzymes** have also proven themselves. These are the same as the enzymes produced by the pancreas – just in tablet form. These pancreatic enzymes support the process of breaking down the food and in turn help the intestine. Besides, they take the burden off the pancreas, which gives it a chance to regenerate itself.

Furthermore, everyday life has a big impact on the well-being of the pancreas. **Alcohol and stress** above all are very hard on the pancreas. If the laboratory tests show that the pancreas is not working well enough, then it is necessary to reduce alcohol consumption as well as stress significantly.

3.9 Stress

In seeking for the cause of digestive disorders, we are now moving somewhat away from the organs and moving towards the nerves and hormones. Ultimately, physical and psychological levels are very closely interwoven. If something happens on one level, it always has an impact on the other level.

The interconnection between psychological strain and IBS might be difficult to understand at first glance. One of them seems to happen in the head, the other one in the intestine. In theory, these two processes are spatially separated and seem to have little to do with each other. Well, if only it were that simple. As we have meanwhile seen, everything in the body is connected to each other.

Of course, you can ignore this relationship and simply assert: "Your state of mind has no influence on the intestine, they are two separate things." However, in that case you shouldn't be surprised if you don't make much progress along the path to healing. The body doesn't really care whether we believe in certain interrelationships or not – it strictly follows the physical, biological and chemical principles of nature. It is similar to gravity on Earth. Gravity doesn't care at all whether we believe in it or not. It is there and has an impact on everyone – regardless of whether they believe in it or not!

In the intestine, there are **millions (!) of nerve cells** and this is the reason why the intestine is also called the second brain.

It contains a huge network of neuronal connections and these intestinal nerve cells constantly communicate with the nerves in the brain. Therefore, stress or conflicts can impact the intestine quite quickly. To get a better understanding, let's take a closer look at all that happens in the intestine under stress and psychological strain.

Stress played a very important role in evolution: It prepares us for an extreme physical situation – either to escape or to attack. The development from the great apes to modern humans took several million years. During this time, we were constantly exposed to dangers in nature and only those who escaped from these dangers time and again were able to survive. The less successful species, on the other hand, became extinct. We are true survivors and our body comprises the most proven survival mechanisms over millions of years.

This means, our body is thus completely tuned for survival. We have already looked at what happens to the body in a life-threatening or stressful situation in the example with the saber-toothed tiger. In such a situation, the body needs salts and high-energy substances as quickly as possible. In the end, it must be able to act immediately or run for a long distance.

In order to survive, the body taps into all its energy supplies. Sources like fat contain big amounts of energy, but they are not available immediately. In such a stressful situation, the body uses any food that is still in the intestine – even if it is not fully digested yet. The tight junctions (the gap between two cells in the intestinal wall) become wider. The intestinal wall consequently gets more permeable overall and as a result, the energy-rich substances needed for fleeing are absorbed more quickly. The body deliberately provokes an "artificial" leaky gut in order to survive.

If the stress now becomes permanent, the intestinal wall remains permeable. This is because the body in fact does not know that stress nowadays has nothing to do with the struggle for survival. When the brain sends the message "stress," the body doesn't ask whether the stress comes from your boss, from conflicts with other people or from a saber-toothed tiger. It gets ready for a fight or to escape every time – just as it has already done very successfully for the past millions of years.

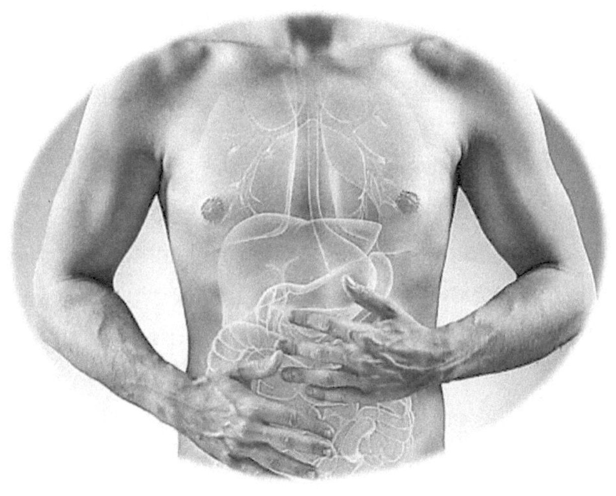

These correlations clearly show how constant stress can lead to IBS. If you are under stress, not only do the "tight junctions" in the intestine expand, but the body also releases hormones and messenger substances. For some hormones, even the smallest quantities of a trillionth of a gram are sufficient to trigger a reaction in the body [12].

In most cases, the messenger substances are released by the immune system. But how does our body know when it should release the messenger substances? Any kind of external stimuli can cause this reaction and one crucial signal for this to happen is stress. Besides, messenger substances are involved in inflammatory reactions everywhere in the body: Be it in case of an autoimmune disease or an inflamed intestine. This sets off the following chain reaction: Stress leads to the release of messenger substances – these in turn lead to inflammations – and these inflammations make the intestine permeable.

How to measure stress?

To determine what exactly happens in the body under stress, the neurophysiologist Professor Dirk Hellhammer carried out an interesting experiment. He had participants take part in a stress test and at the same time he measured the stress level in their body. It turned out that some participants did not experience the entire test as stressful at all, although their physical stress values rose to dizzying heights [13]. The perception of stress and the actual reaction of the body can therefore be very different. Even if you aren't under massive stress due to a deadline or feeling rushed all the time, it is still worth taking a closer look at your own psychological environment if you suffer from digestive problems.

Stress can be measured using many different values, such as by the stress hormone cortisol in saliva, by the messenger substances serotonin and interleukin, by enzymes such as alpha-amylase or by heart rate variability (HRV). The question here is: How meaningful are these values and how well do they reflect everyday psychological strain?

However, you don't have to bring out the big guns by using extensive stress tests made in the laboratory. It would make more sense to first of all get a sense of whether stress has any effect at all on your intestinal symptoms. The following two questions might help:

Do your symptoms become significantly better during stress-free times, such as vacation?

Do your symptoms get worse during very stressful times?

Stress and anxiety always have a certain impact on the intestine. You can see that already from the saying: "Someone soils their pants from fear." If you don't notice any improvement in your intestinal disorders even during a long, relaxing vacation, then stress is probably not the main reason for the digestive problems. On the other hand, the situation is different if your symptoms improve significantly during more relaxed phases or if they worsen under severe stress.

What can you do about stress?

If you suspect that stress is responsible for your digestive problems, there are many potential ways to do something about it. Basically, there are two important starting points: The incoming stress should be significantly reduced and you should create a balance to everyday hustle and bustle.

The first and most important step is of course to reduce stress, because even the best relaxation exercises are of little use if you are constantly experiencing a lot of new tension on a daily basis. Then you are always just running after the problem. Of course, it isn't possible to eliminate all the major sources of stress overnight, but a lot can be done over the long term. The most difficult step is usually to get off the everyday stress hamster wheel, to analyze yourself and to even perceive the stress which has become part of everyday life.

The second step is to create a good mental balance in order to balance out stressful everyday life. There are several options available to do this, such as **meditation, progressive muscle relaxation or autogenic training**. Even simply a few minutes of silence during the day or a walk in the woods can create a wonderful balance.

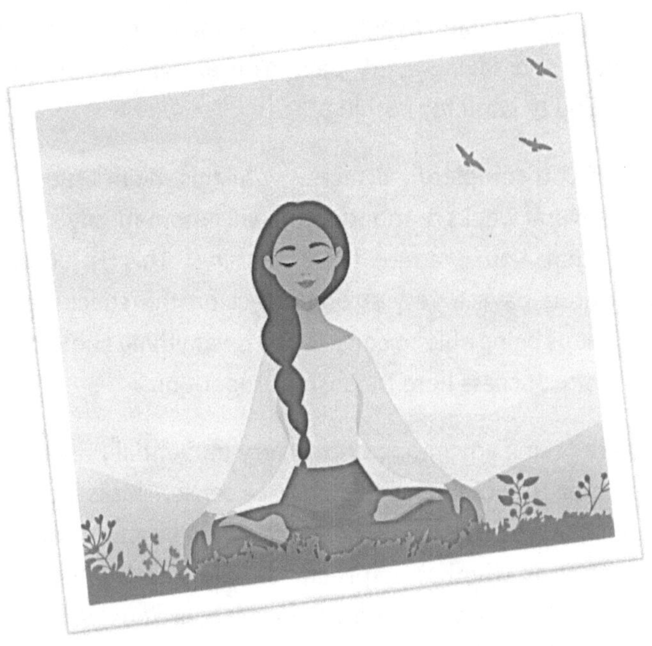

However, tension and stress don't just necessarily come from the outside, they can also be "homemade" due to your own thoughts. In this context, especially self-confidence plays a crucial role. People with low self-esteem take things much more to heart or often blame themselves for mistakes. Of course, these are not good preconditions for reducing stress.

To significantly improve self-confidence, "**positive affirmations**" have really shown their worth. Although this term is rather awkward, it means nothing more than saying short, clearly worded sentences to yourself. Through the constant repetition, the message penetrates deep into the subconscious. This principle can be illustrated very well using a reverse example. Imagine a little man sitting on your shoulder and saying every day: "You are weak. You are a loser. You're good for nothing."

Even if you completely disagree with this mean little man, after several weeks or months you will automatically start to think that you are good for nothing. This is because repetitions have a very strong effect on the subconscious without us being able to consciously do anything about it. So, the key to success here is constant repetition.

We are taking advantage of this very influential principle of repetition, but of course in a positive sense. This is intended to build up your own self-confidence, step by step. It doesn't matter at all whether you really believe in this principle of positive affirmations or not: Your subconscious will simply believe what is being said at some point, due to the daily repetitions. In the event of more serious or traumatizing issues, you should take advantage of support from a trained therapist in addition to these measures. Psychotherapists have the necessary theoretical knowledge and besides this, they deal with patients who have similar problems on a daily basis. This enables them to draw on a wealth of psychological experience.

Info-Box 

- ✓ There are millions of nerve cells in the intestine and they are very closely linked to the brain (intestine-brain axis)
- ✓ In situations of stress or fear, the body deliberately gives itself a leaky gut, so that it can get to the food in the intestine quickly. For a short time, this self-generated leaky gut is very useful
- ✓ If stress or anxiety persists over a longer time, then the digestive disorders will remain
- ✓ What can you do about it? First, find the cause of the stress/fear and remove it, while making sure you get to relax at the same time (with positive affirmations, meditation or autogenic training)

3.10 Summary: The best treatment methods

In the previous chapters, we took a closer look at the causes and the resulting treatment options for IBS. With so many different options and all the medical terms, you can quickly lose sight of the essentials: *Which treatment is important? And what is the best way to start?*

In order to tackle the most important things first, I have briefly summarized the most important measures in this chapter. Beforehand, there are three points that are so important for a successful treatment that I would like to emphasize them once again here.

1.) The difference between cause and symptom

Anyone who really wants to get rid of their digestive problems permanently has to ask this crucial question: What is the cause of the disease and what is only a symptom? Symptoms are all the **noticeable and visible consequences** of an illness like flatulence, abdominal pain, itchy skin, diarrhea and much more. The cause, on the other hand, is the real reason for the disease. It is often hidden and cannot be seen or felt in any way.

But even if it is hidden, the cause is crucial and it is the linchpin of the disease. If the cause disappears, then the annoying symptoms disappear automatically. It just doesn't work the other way around: You can deal with the symptoms for as long and intensively as you like, but the cause won´t go away.

The difference between cause and symptom is in itself not very complicated. Especially physicians who have studied medicine for a long time should actually have deeply internalized this difference, because the entire further treatment for the patient depends on that.

It is all the more incomprehensible to me that when it comes to the topics of irritable bowel syndrome, food intolerances or histamine intolerance, a very large group of doctors only concentrate on suppressing the symptoms. In the past, I have spoken to a large number of people who have digestive problems and received responses from readers. Almost all of them tried a lot of different things and consulted their doctor. Unfortunately, the doctors' approach was in almost all cases only symptom-oriented.

Also, with IBS and medicine in general, money plays a big role nowadays. When you have someone with IBS and you were to go straight for the root causes, then a very large percentage of patients could be fully healed. These people wouldn´t have to come back for endless treatments or buy medicine for years.

On the other hand, if there is only a suppression of the symptoms, the patient has to come again and again for years or even decades. Laboratories, doctors and pharmacies earn a decent amount of money from someone who will have to come back regularly. However, there are just no earnings from healthy people.

We can only hope that there will be a rethinking in the future – it would be very beneficial for all the patients!

2.) First the diagnosis – then the treatment

In most cases, digestive disorders usually start to show up as unpleasant symptoms. Something or other is pinching, pushing, or bloating and just doesn't feel right anymore. At some point you realize that you have to become active and here, most people make a big mistake by just taking "something" for their digestive problems.

From emergency drops for an irritable bowel, bloating relievers or tablets for diarrhea, it's all available. They are not all bad medications, but in most cases, there is no permanent improvement when you take them. You can try it out yourself: When you stop taking them, the problems will come back.

You took some medicine, which is made exactly for your digestive problems, but you didn´t get any better – why is that? Simply, because there was no testing done to determine exactly what the underlying problem is. There are several thousand medicines for "digestive disorders." If you just wanted to try out all the medications indiscriminately, you would have to live for at least 150 years.

The variety of medicine is really wide: There are special remedies for inflammation, for candida fungal infection, for a lack of gut bacteria or a weakened pancreas. As you can see already: There are a whole lot of starting points. That is why it is so enormously important to first get the right laboratory test and only then take targeted action against it. One of the most important rules is therefore: "First the diagnosis – then the treatment!" First you have to test and only then you can take the medicine.

Therefore, I recommend to start with a comprehensive stool sample, a test for vitamins and minerals as well as a heavy metal test. This gives you clarity and sends you in exactly the right direction – namely in the direction of a healthy gut.

3.) Listen to your own body

Let´s take an example: If you want to find out if you are intolerant of certain foods, there are many tests for this. But it is not the test that decides whether you really can tolerate the food, but rather it is your body alone. If the test says that you can handle milk products very well, but you are always getting sick after having milk products, then you should rather listen to your body instead of the test.

It is only your body that decides if a treatment will ultimately work for you and it is very important to listen to your inner self and pay attention to the signals from your own body.

Basically, I recommend taking the following steps for a therapy for IBS, in this order:

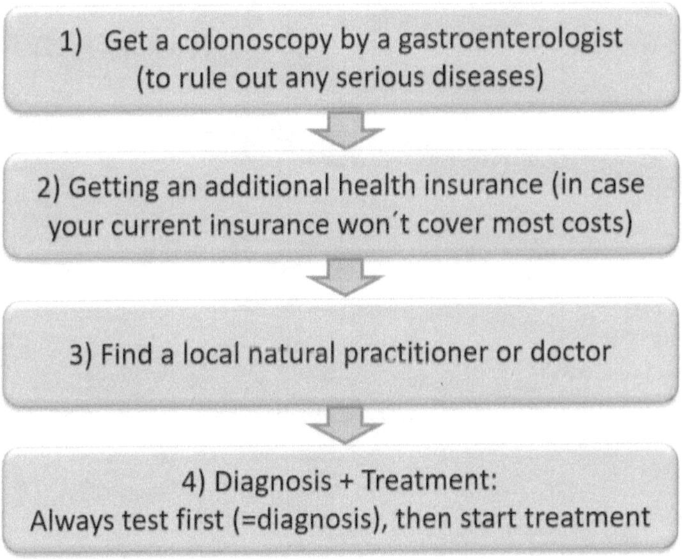

1) Get a colonoscopy by a gastroenterologist (to rule out any serious diseases)

↓

2) Getting an additional health insurance (in case your current insurance won´t cover most costs)

↓

3) Find a local natural practitioner or doctor

↓

4) Diagnosis + Treatment:
Always test first (=diagnosis), then start treatment

You don´t want to just get fine laboratory values on paper, but rather the ultimate goal is to heal the physical problems! Even if laboratory values are very reliable nowadays, they nevertheless only provide a reference point or an orientation. It is of no use to you if you improve a bad laboratory value enormously, but still have the same symptoms or the pain just did not go away. In this case, the value on paper will have changed for you, but you are still struggling with the symptoms. In the end, no laboratory can tell you if you are healed or not – this, only your body can tell you.

Finding the cause of IBS is not simple and the **causes** can be very different in each person. In summary, the following are the points to be addressed:

	Possible cause	How to test for it?	
Food intolerances	**Histamine**	"DAO value" and "total histamine value" in blood (test twice, they can fluctuate)	✓
	Lactose intolerance	Hydrogen breath test for lactose	✓
	Fructose intolerance	Hydrogen breath test for fructose	✓
	Gluten intolerance	Blood test for: - Transglutaminase – IgA - Endomysium-IgA - Total-IgA	✓
Underlying causes	**Disturbed intestinal flora**	Testing bifidobacteria and lactobacilli in a stool sample	✓
	Vitamins and Minerals	Check the status of your vitamins and minerals (only in whole blood, not in serum)	✓
	Heavy metals	Chelate infusions (with DMSA and EDTA)	✓
	Pancreatic weakness	"Pancreatic elastase value" in stool sample (test at least twice)	✓
	HPU-Test (metabolic	HPU value in 24 hour urine (alternative is KPU test)	✓
	Small intestinal bact. overgrowth (SIBO)	Breath test with lactulose	✓
	Taking hormones (e.g. the pill, coil)	Do the digestion symptoms improve after you stop taking the hormones?	✓
	Stress	Do the symptoms improve during times of relaxation or worsen under stress?	✓

Table 2: Causes for IBS and methods to test them.

4 SOS medicine

IBS often comes with the typical digestive problems like diarrhea, constipation, loud abdominal noises, pain or flatulence. These symptoms can impose significant limits on everyday life and can be physically and mentally very stressful. However, these symptoms do not just appear randomly; they are always only a consequence of something being wrong in the body.

The body does not express its problems and worries in words, but uses symptoms as its language. It is not always easy to interpret the language of the body correctly. However, the better you learn to understand it, all the faster the body can recover.

To heal the cause of a disease, it usually takes some time to reach this goal. For you to be able to live as symptom-free as possible during this time, there are some good emergency measures in case your gut causes serious problems.

4.1 Flatulence

Even in healthy people, it is completely normal for fermentation processes and gases to occur in the intestine. Flatulence is something completely natural and does not always automatically indicate a disease. Rather decisive is how often the flatulence occurs during the day and whether it is perceived as annoying.

A certain proportion of the air in the intestine reaches the lungs via the blood and is exhaled there. That is a process that we don´t even notice. You can say that flatulence occurring about 10 to 15 times per day can be considered normal. That means, once per hour. Only if you regularly suffer from severe flatulence, pain or other ailments occur along with it, should you take appropriate countermeasures.

There are basically two reasons for flatulence: **Nutritional as well as organic reasons**. Nutritional causes include all food, drink or behavior patterns that cause flatulence even in healthy people.

Some foods are well known to cause increased development of gas in the intestine. These are for example:

- Certain types of vegetables such as onions, leeks or cabbage
- Mushrooms
- Eggs
- Pulses such as beans or lentils
- Freshly baked bread

One reason for developing more gas in the intestine when you eat certain foods is that they contain a high proportion of indigestible fiber. Anyone who is generally prone to increased flatulence should therefore avoid these foods in order to avoid further strain on the intestine and the entire organism.

Dietary fiber is generally considered healthy and is often recommended for a balanced diet and this holds true for healthy people. On the other hand, if the digestive system is already damaged and you are suffering from flatulence anyway, then you should avoid fiber, because it puts an additional strain on the intestine.

Also, sugar substitutes such as sorbitol, maltitol or xylitol can cause flatulence. These substances are often found in "sugar-free" lemonade, chewing gum, diet sweets and any "light" products which declare they are sugar-free. Besides fiber-rich food and sugar-free products, any kind of food intolerance like histamine, lactose, fructose or gluten can reinforce flatulence.

Beyond food, there is more that can lead to a bloated stomach. Certain eating habits also promote gas formation in the intestine:

- Eating late or just before going to sleep
- Eating too quickly and not chewing food well
- Eating portions that are too large
- Too many different foods in one meal
- Carbonated drinks

If flatulence keeps occurring again and again, regardless of your diet, then the causes are more likely to be organic. In this case, you should take a closer look above all at the **pancreas** (*Chapter 3.8)* as well as the **intestinal flora** (*Chapter 3.3*).

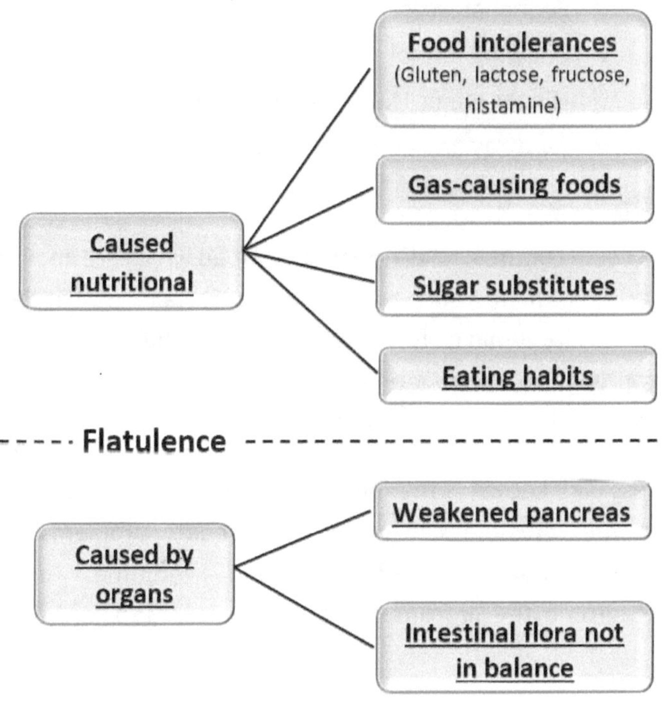

Especially identifying food intolerances is not that easy, but once you have determined what your body cannot digest well, then you can achieve a lot through diet alone. To do something against flatulence, three measures can bring very good results in the long term: Pepping up the intestinal flora, checking for a weakness of the pancreas and identifying food intolerances.

However, if you want to do something about flatulence in the short term, there are some good and natural remedies. The following remedies have proven very successful:

- √ Fennel-anise-caraway tea
- √ Chewing fennel seeds
- √ Ginger tea or freshly prepared ginger
- √ Caraway and cumin seeds as spices in food

In some cultures, when meals are served which are known to cause flatulence, such as lentil dishes, certain anti-flatulence spices like cumin or fennel are added already when the food is prepared. Exercise or a digestive walk have also proven valuable in case of excess flatulence.

Less well known is the fact that excessive gas accumulation in the intestine can even cause heart problems. This phenomenon is called "Roemheld syndrome." In this syndrome, the air from the abdomen presses so hard against the diaphragm that it can impact the entire chest as well as the heart.

Constant flatulence can severely limit the quality of life and it is an attempt by the body to convey in its own language that something is wrong and should be corrected.

Info-Box 

✓ **Nutritional causes:**

- Food intolerances
- Flatulence-causing foods (like legumes, cabbage vegetables, whole grains etc.)
- Check your nutritional and eating habits (e.g. eating too fast)
- Sugar substitutes can cause flatulence. They are often used in "light" products and named "sorbitol", "maltitol" or "xylitol"

✓ **Organic causes:**

- Intestinal flora
- Pancreas

✓ **Measures:**

- Fennel-anis-caraway tea
- Plenty of exercise (digestive walk)
- Ginger, Parsley
- Caraway and cumin used as spice in food

4.2 Diarrhea

There are usually two major causes for diarrhea. In some cases, pathogens like bacteria and viruses are behind it. Besides pathogens, diarrhea could also be a defense reaction of the body. This can happen in case of a food intolerance or when the bowel is generally irritated and inflamed.

Especially when travelling, a bacterial infection is the most common cause of diarrhea. The body is usually not familiar with the bacterial world you find in the destination country. The worse the hygienic standards in the country, the greater the chance of getting diarrhea. However, even in the familiar home environment, gastrointestinal infections are also common.

The most important thing is to find the **cause of the infection**. For example, if you were eating at a restaurant and you got diarrhea afterwards, then this only involves a one-time matter. But if you continue to consume contaminated water or spoiled food daily, then new pathogens will be introduced to the body over and over again and the diarrhea persists. Therefore, it is absolutely necessary to check whether the **source of the infection** has already been eliminated or not.

To help the body remove the bacteria as quickly as possible, there are many good remedies, which have the property of binding bacteria and toxins. These include:

- √ Activated charcoal (mostly in tablet form)
- √ Psyllium seed husks
- √ Medicinal clay

Another good treatment for diarrhea is consuming gut bacteria and yeast cultures. These products are usually available in pharmacies and they can suppress the bacteria that cause sickness in the intestine as well as calm down the entire intestinal tract.

In case of an infection, it is extremely important to get rid of the bacteria or viruses as quickly as possible. Therefore, you should be particularly careful with so-called peristaltic inhibitors (such as "*loperamide*"). These medications slow down the peristaltic movement a lot, which leads to the situation that the pathogenic bacteria or viruses remain in the body. The intestine has to keep fighting against these invaders and it cannot calm down. Therefore, a peristaltic inhibitor should be used carefully and only as a last option, when other measures didn´t work.

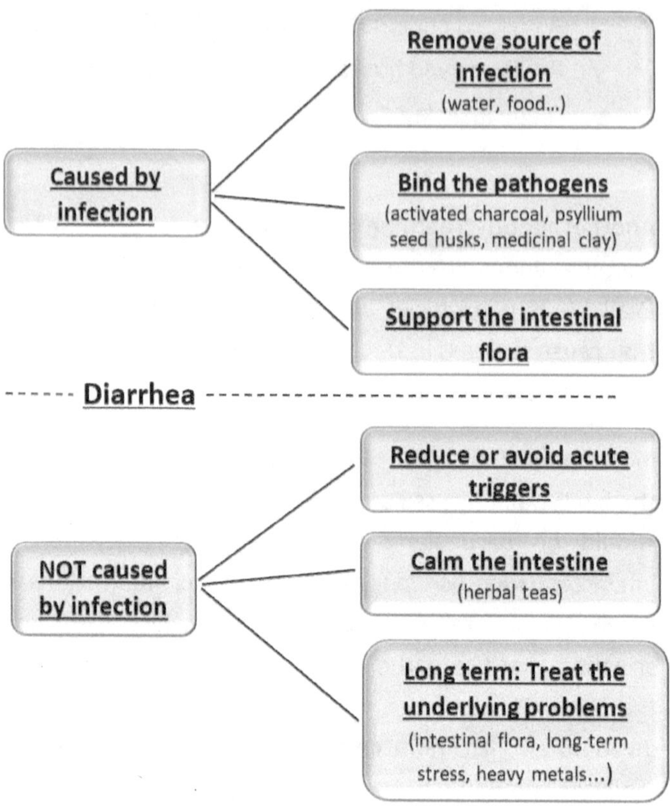

When diarrhea occurs not from an infection but rather comes from a general defense reaction in the body, the focus should not be on removing bacteria, but on calming the intestine down. The next step is then to find the reason why the body reacts to certain influences or circumstances with diarrhea.

Diarrhea can be a defense reaction in case of:

- √ Food intolerances
- √ Psychological stress
- √ Intestinal flora is out of balance
- √ Heavy metal toxicity
- √ Inflammation of the intestinal mucosa
- √ A side effect from medications

If diarrhea keeps coming back and no pathogens are involved, then you have to start looking for the reason that makes the body react like this. One main reason for regular diarrhea can be a food intolerance as well as severe stress and psychological strain. If the diarrhea improves a lot during times that are more peaceful or when you are on vacation, this can be a first indication that stress is the trigger.

However, curing the deeper lying causes for diarrhea will definitely take some time. In the short run, you can use some herbs to feel better and help the intestine to calm down. Especially herbal teas like blackberry and raspberry leaves as well as St. John's wort have proven their worth. These remedies have an astringent effect. This gently slows down the peristaltic movement. Drinking chamomile tea can also help to calm down an upset intestine.

In addition to the measures mentioned, which mainly work in the intestine, it is necessary to make up for water and electrolyte loss. When you have diarrhea, the body loses large quantities of water and minerals. This often shows up as exhaustion and tiredness. Therefore, it is necessary to have a high fluid intake of more than two liters per day, even if you feel weakened and you aren´t thirsty. To replenish your electrolyte balance after an episode of diarrhea, electrolyte solutions from the pharmacy, a diet rich in vital substances and minerals, as well as salty beverages or food are all especially effective.

On the other hand, it is important to avoid certain foods and beverages when you suffer from diarrhea, since they will irritate the intestine even more:

- Caffeine
- Alcohol
- Black tea
- Sugary beverages
- Milk and dairy products
- Foods you don't tolerate
- Very spicy dishes

It is also advisable to eat a bland diet during the diarrhea phase and for some time afterwards. This is because the intestine should be able to recover to some extent from its previous exertions and use its energy for the healing process.

Suitable for a bland diet are:

- √ Apple grated with its peel
- √ Mashed bananas
- √ Vegetable soups
- √ Boiled or pureed vegetables

Info-Box 

✓ **General:**

- Make up for water and electrolyte loss
- Bland diet
- Avoid irritating foods and beverages

✓ **If caused by pathogens (bacteria or virus):**

- Find the source of the infection (e.g. contaminated water or spoiled food)
- Remove pathogens from your body with activated charcoal, psyllium seed husks or medicinal clay
- Building up the intestinal flora with gut bacteria like E. coli bacteria or yeast cultures

✓ **If NOT caused by bacteria or virus:**

- ✓ Find the cause (stress, food intolerance ...)
- ✓ Herbal teas (blackberry, raspberry leaves, St. John's wort)

4.3 Constipation

Constipation is the opposite reaction to diarrhea. While with diarrhea the body wants to get rid of something, with constipation it is clinging on to something. Constipation can have physical as well as psychological reasons.

If the constipation comes from physical causes, then the peristaltic movement is usually too slow. At the same time, a general sluggishness in everyday life usually has a reflective effect on the intestine. Therefore, daily exercise is very important for people who are prone to constipation.

Adequate hydration is also an important point when you are constipated. The large intestine removes water from the chyme (semiliquid food mass), but if the body has the feeling that it gets too little fluid, then it tries to extract as much fluid as possible.

Since humans consist of more than 70% water, adequate hydration is very important. When you drink enough and the body receives the signal that it will be supplied with enough fluid, then it is no longer so urgently dependent on the fluid in the intestine. As a rule of thumb, the liquid intake should be at least 1.5 liters per day for a good hydration.

Besides this, consuming an adequate supply of dietary fiber is very important to prevent constipation. You can get a good amount of fiber from eating whole grains, fruits and vegetables, if you can tolerate them. Furthermore, fiber can also be supplemented by certain products such as linseed, psyllium seed husks or bran.

When supplementing fiber, it is very important to drink plenty of fluids with it. These fiber supplements bulk up in the intestine and the stool volume increases. This exerts pressure on the intestinal wall and gives the body a signal to empty itself and this is exactly what you need when you are constipated. However, if you drink too few fluids along with these fiber-rich bulking agents, the constipation can even get worse.

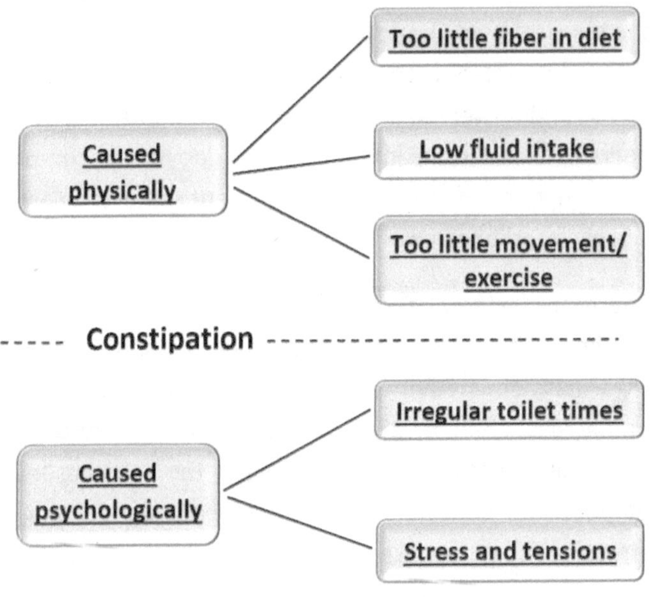

Another important aspect is to have a regulated lifestyle and especially a regular time to go to the toilet. This gives the body the opportunity to adjust to certain processes in terms of time. Furthermore, medications can also be responsible for constipation. If the constipation occurred after starting on a certain medication, then this medication might be a possible cause. If the constipation was there beforehand, then it is very unlikely that the medication is the cause. Also, the hormonal balance can have a major impact on being constipated, especially for women.

In addition to these physical causes, it can also be the case that you become constipated due to psychological stress. Even though this topic is usually more difficult to grasp than the physical level, your state of mind plays an important role here. The intestine consists of an enormously large nerve plexus and bowel movement is primarily controlled by these nerves. However, the intestinal nerves do not act completely independently of their environment, but rather they are very closely interlinked with our brain.

Therefore, external psychological influences have an impact on peristaltic movement and that happens completely regardless of whether we want it to or not. In principle, this bodily reaction makes a lot of sense and is very useful. During the millennia of human development, the body has learned to adapt its behavior to the corresponding situations. In stressful situations, like fleeing from wild animals, surviving is the top priority while digestion is of no importance at all in such a situation.

In stressful situations, all our energy will therefore be bundled together for tasks that are necessary for escape or defense. When stressful situations arise nowadays, then the body also switches into this attack or flight mode and greatly reduces its digestive performance. It was and is essential for survival that the body becomes constipated in tense situations.

If any kind of stress was always bad for us, then every single high-level manager or CEO would become sick sooner or later, but this is not the case. Of course, not every little bit of stress is bad for the intestine. It's more a matter of permanent stress and if the stress is perceived as negative. The decisive factor in analyzing your own stress level is not to compare whether someone else is under much more stress than you are, but whether you perceive your own situation as being under strain and as stressful.

The major step here is to understand that certain physical processes are set off in stressful situations and that they cannot simply be switched off. Accordingly, it is necessary to reduce stress as much as possible in your personal and professional environment. This is always easier said than done, but your intestine and general health will thank you for it.

One problematic matter for treating constipation is when you are using laxative medications over a longer period of time. As a result, the body forgets the feeling of how to empty itself naturally and on its own. At some point, going to the toilet becomes dependent on the medication. While taking laxative medication, the root causes of the constipation, such as a lack of fluid, other medications or stress, are still present. The dose has to be constantly increased and you keep distancing yourself more and more from the natural state of digestion.

As with many other physical symptoms, the best thing to do for constipation is to try out which measures are most effective for you. If you have two patients who both are constipated, one measure can have great success for one person, while in contrast the same measure has no effect at all for the other person.

Info-Box 

✓ **Find the cause:**

- Psychological strain (holding on to something)
- Medications
- Lack of fluid

✓ **Measures:**

- Plenty of exercise
- Increase fluid intake (drink more than 1.5 liters water or tea a day)
- Taking dietary fiber

4.4 Loud abdominal noises

Even if loud abdominal noises and gurgling in the intestine aren't that dramatic, these symptoms can become a serious psychological strain. This is especially true if you are sitting in meetings, in a waiting room or in quiet spaces with other people. When it comes to abdominal noises, we must first distinguish between stomach noises and intestinal noises.

It isn't always possible to clearly distinguish where the abdominal noises come from. Sounds that come from your stomach can be associated with being hungry, feeling "stuffed" or belching. Intestinal noise come from somewhat deeper in the abdominal cavity, although it isn't always easy to make a clear distinction because the stomach and intestine are very close to each other in some places.

If the abdominal gurgling is from the intestine, then there are often two causes to be considered. The noise can either be caused by a build-up of air or it can be noise from peristaltic movement. If the cause is air in the abdomen, then you can apply all the measures that are listed in *Chapter 4.1 Flatulence*.

For food intolerances, in the beginning it isn't that easy to figure out which foods might cause the flatulence. With histamine intolerance, the symptoms can come shortly after a meal, but they may also appear the next day. If you have consumed beverages or liquid foods, the length of time in the stomach is significantly shorter and they pass through very quickly.

With solid food, most meals remain in the stomach for a long time and it takes some hours before they even arrive in the intestine. The stomach needs this time to pre-digest the food well. With such a long digestion time, it can take up to 24 hours before the flatulence shows up. That means that the time between eating certain foods and flatulence showing up can vary from a few minutes up to a whole day.

When you have figured out that you have too much air in the abdomen, then you again need to find the root cause for this. To get started, I would first take a closer look at the pancreas, the intestinal flora and, of course, at food intolerances.

Peristaltic movement can be another cause of loud abdominal noises. The intestine constantly keeps the bolus, which is a "porridge" of chewed food, moving on in order to excrete it at the end. There is a constant muscular movement in the intestine and for all muscle movements in the body to run smoothly, the presence of **magnesium** is particularly important.

Magnesium is also very important for athletes or for people who get frequent muscle cramps. The requirements of the muscles in the intestine are similar: The intestinal muscles cannot function optimally without enough magnesium. Therefore, taking magnesium supplements can be very helpful if you suffer from loud abdominal noises. However, not just the amount of magnesium per tablet is important, but also the chemical compound. The most common chemical compounds on the market are magnesium chelate, magnesium citrate or magnesium carbonate.

From the ingredient list, it is easy to see which form of magnesium is used in a product. Carbonate compounds are in general not advisable, and not only for magnesium. These bind to a lot of gastric acid and thus weaken a very important digestive organ. This in turn has an impact on the intestine as things proceed. Citrate and chelate compounds are significantly better for the stomach. The advantage of chelates in particular is their very high bioavailability.

When you take a tablet with 100 mg of magnesium, the body does not generally absorb the full 100 mg, but only a certain portion of it. The better the chemical compound, the better the body can absorb the magnesium. However, you should be careful with too much substitution of magnesium, since an overdose can lead to diarrhea or other side effects.

If the intestine is generally irritated or inflamed, then spicy food and fiery spices can also cause noises. Of course, a certain spiciness really peps up the food, but this great taste experience unfortunately doesn't do much good when your intestine suffers from it later on. Therefore, too spicy food can also be a cause for loud intestinal noise and very spicy food should in general be avoided when you are struggling with digestive disorders.

Info-Box

✓ **Measures:**

- Too much air can be a cause -> see Flatulence
- Supplement magnesium
- Supplement multi-vitamin compounds
- Avoid spicy foods and fiery spices
- Check for candida fungus infection

5 Nothing doing without money – Supplemental health insurance

It would be great to start immediately with the treatment of IBS, but unfortunately there is still a catch to the whole thing – and that is, as so often, our dear friend money.

The basic problems that patients face are mostly the same: Your doctor couldn´t help you with the standard treatment methods and now you have to start looking for a solution to your digestive disorders on your own.

Since the "normal" methods got you nowhere, you have to think outside the box. Unfortunately, everything outside the box is generally not paid for by regular health insurance and you are usually responsible for the costs yourself.

Most health insurance companies only cover certain services and, of course, the vast majority of IBS treatments are not among them. Even if a doctor prescribes certain laboratory tests or treatments, the patients must pay for everything which is not in the standard catalog of services.

However, the interest in additional services has increased enormously in recent years. Since a majority of doctors do not offer any treatment for IBS, most patients go to a natural practitioner. Private insurance companies have recognized this opportunity and in many cases expanded coverage for certain treatments or they introduced additional health insurance for services by natural practitioners.

Health insurance coverage and choices vary widely by country, and even by plan within each country. A comprehensive review of coverage options is beyond the scope of this book. However, I would like to give you an example from Germany (where I live), showing how difficult it is for patients here not to end up being responsible for the costs all by themselves. In Germany, having health insurance is obligatory, so every citizen is covered by health insurance and that's a really good thing. For the insurance, there are two options: Most people are enrolled in a statutory health insurance company and those who can afford it are privately insured.

Meanwhile, there are hundreds of supplementary insurance plans and it takes a while to work your way through the large selection. However, this is great for patients here, since they finally have an option that can provide coverage for a large part of the costs. A few years ago, this option did not exist at all and patients had to cover the costs all on their own.

Most supplemental insurance plans here cover a large number of laboratory tests and treatment services that are not covered by standard health insurance. The only little downside of the supplementary insurance is that there is a maximum limit for each year and most of them cover only 80% of the costs.

However, from the insurer's point of view, the 80% limit makes a lot of sense. If the insurance company would cover 100% of the costs, many insured persons would take advantage of services that they actually don't really need –

just because they are free of charge. So, when insured persons participate by paying even just 20% of the cost, it makes sure that the patients only use treatments that are necessary.

In summary, it makes sense to check first with your health insurance if they cover certain IBS treatments. If they don´t cover it, then searching for additional health insurance options is a good idea. When you obtain extra coverage, you don´t have to use it for the rest of your life. Most contracts are for one or two years and can be cancelled when the insurance is not needed anymore.

For the entire IBS treatment, there are several ways to keep costs within a reasonable range:

- √ Check with your own health insurance company if they cover the required services for IBS
- √ If not, try to find appropriate supplementary insurance (if available and cost-effective)
- √ Taxes: It makes sense to check, if services rendered are possibly tax-deductible
- √ If nothing has helped: Ask your health insurance provider for a reimbursement afterwards and an individual case decision

6 FAQ – The most important questions about IBS at a glance

Where did I get my IBS from?

Hmm, that is a difficult question, because there can be a lot of different reasons for every person. For some patients, it started with antibiotic treatment, which disrupted everything in their intestinal flora and unpleasant contemporaries were able to spread through the intestine.

For others, it could be that heavy metal toxicity is behind it, which blocks many important cell processes in the body. The digestive problems could also come from taking medication over a long time, or it may be due to HPU metabolic disorder and so on. As you can see: There are a lot of ways to catch this pleasant IBS.

I have digestive problems all the time. What should I do first?

Unfortunately, it isn't easy to identify the cause of digestive disorders just by the symptoms. Here, the best way to start is with a stool sample that is sent to a laboratory.

Once you have sent a stool sample to the laboratory, I would definitely recommend having multiple values tested right away. This is because just one or two value alone don´t say much about the general condition of your intestine. The puzzle can only be put together by using several values. After you have all the laboratory values from the stool sample together, a reasonable treatment plan can then be drawn up on this basis. The most important laboratory values for IBS include the pH value, gut bacteria, alpha-1 antitrypsin, sIgA, calprotectin, candida and molds, as well as pancreatic elastase. Parallel to the stool sample, I would recommend to check for food intolerances. Avoiding intolerant foods might sound simple, but it can make a big change for IBS patients.

I got the results from my stool sample. What can I do now?

When treating IBS, there are several points from where you can start. The most important factor is to find out which foods you can´t tolerate and to avoid them. Another good starting point is to feed the intestinal flora with "good" bacteria from probiotic supplements. For some people, this already might be enough to get their digestive disorders under control. Just be aware, that none of the treatments will work within two or three days. It takes some time for the body to get things back in order.

However, sometimes, the trigger for your IBS is still in the body. Then this trigger has to be tracked down. To do this, there are several starting points that have helped many other patients: Checking for heavy metals, for food intolerances, for HPU metabolic disorder, too much stress or a weakened pancreas.

The best testing and treatment options are listed in *Chapter 3* and described in detail there. This is where the detective search for the cause should begin.

How can I find a good doctor or therapist?

The first step for most people with IBS is usually to consult their family doctor or a general practitioner. If he or she can´t do anything about your digestive disorders, then at this point, it is time to search for alternatives.

However, it is not that easy to find someone who is specialized in treating IBS patients. In many countries, there are certain therapist platforms on the Internet nowadays, where you can search for a specialist in your area or the next big city. The big advantage of such Internet sites is that they offer ratings about the therapists. That's a great chance to see how happy other patients were with the therapist before you make an appointment there.

Another important point is that you shouldn´t just search for graduate medical doctors. Natural practitioners in particular have a good approach towards the search for the causes of a disease and can be a good alternative.

Do I have to change my diet?

A change in diet is very important if you have digestive problems, so that the body can recover. Food intolerances keep irritating the intestine anew all the time. There are very reliable tests to determine certain food intolerances. In any case, tests should be done for gluten, lactose (milk sugar), fructose (fruit sugar) and histamine. More about the right test procedures is described in *Chapter 3.2*.

Closing words

We have now proven one thing: Nobody can claim anymore that nothing can be done about IBS or digestive disorders. There are many good treatment options that focus primarily on the root of the evil. However, you should have some patience, because it can take time before IBS is healed. Experienced therapists calculate that it can take between six months and one year for the intestine to recover. That's a really long time. However, even a treatment that takes longer would still be better than doing nothing at all and just accepting the fact that you have to deal with your digestive problems every day.

You can also expect that there will be high and low phases during the treatment. It's a little like a roller coaster ride. There are days when things go really well and then there are setbacks when you could almost despair. I wish you the ability to remain steadfast and continue on your path, even in difficult times!

And, above all, I hope that these tips have given you a great deal of hope again. You are not alone with your digestive problems and one thing should make you very confident: Many people have made their way back from IBS to a life without any digestive problems at all. A lot is possible, you just need to work hard, go your own way and have some stamina in difficult situations.

Histamine intolerance from a totally new perspective

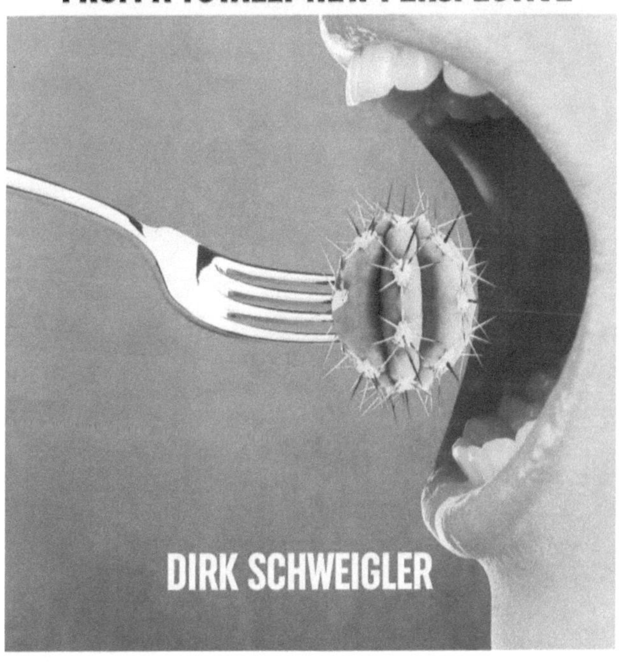

About the author

Dirk Schweigler discovered his passion for writing while he was studying. His diploma thesis was nominated for the *"Friedrich List Prize"* and he has had the opportunity to present his research results at international conferences in Rio de Janeiro as well as in the Netherlands.

Already during his studies, Dirk was fascinated by travel and he backpacked his way several times through Japan, Mexico and the United States. After completing his studies, he wanted to get a new perspective on the world and lived in India for over a year to study the Hindu scriptures. Meanwhile, he has been working as a scientist at a German university hospital for several years now.

Dirk himself was an IBS patient for a long time. Since no doctor could help him anymore, he simply took the healing of his intestinal problems into his own hands. For over three years, he tried out many things, carried out intensive research and exchanged ideas with other patients who were also suffering from digestive disorders. Taking this with him to become an author who distinguishes between the symptoms of a disease and the underlying cause, Dirk is excited to share his findings and prove that "just live with it" is never the answer.

Contact:
Dirk.Schweigler@gmail.com

Bibliography

[1] Wittkamp, P.; Andresen, V.; Broicher, W.; Rose, M.; Burchard, G. D.; Layer, P. et al. (2012): Prävalenz des Reizdarmsyndroms nach den Rom-III-Kriterien in Deutschland und Zusammenhänge mit potentiellen Risikofaktoren. In: *Z Gastroenterol* 50 (08). DOI: 10.1055/s-0032-1323885.

[2] Bayer, W.; Schmid, K. (2013): Gesunder Darm, kranker Darm. Diagnostischer Leitfaden für Darm-assoziierte Erkrankungen. Leinfelden-Echterdingen. Online verfügbar unter http://www.labor-bayer.de/laborinformationen_publikationen/stuhldiagnostik/DrBayer-Gesunder-Darm-kranker-Darm.pdf.

[3] Wittig, F. (2014): Wie Schmerzmittel funktionieren. Hg. v. Südwestrundfunk. Stuttgart. Online verfügbar unter https://www.swr.de/odysso/wie-schmerzmittel-funktionieren/-/id=1046894/did=14623508/nid=1046894/ejo9bs/index.html.

[4] Biovis (2011): Leaky gut. Die erhöhte Durchlässigkeit des Darms – Ursachen und Folgen. Limburg. Online verfügbar unter http://www.biovis.de/resources/Downloads_Aerzte/Aerzte_Fachinfo_DL/Biovis_Leaky_gut_221112.pdf.

[5] Mutter, J.; Haley, B.; Runte, H. (2012): Gesund statt chronisch krank! Der ganzheitliche Weg: Vorbeugung und

Heilung sind möglich. 2. [Aufl.]. Weil der Stadt: Fit-fürs-Leben-Verlag (Gesundheit).

[6] Deutsche Hauptstelle für Suchtfragen e.V. (2018): Alkohol- Zahlen und Fakten. Hamm. Online verfügbar unter http://www.aktionswoche-alkohol.de/fakten-mythen/zahlen-und-fakten/.

[7] Deutsche Gesellschaft für Ernährung (DGE): Referenzwert: Vitamin C. Bonn. Online verfügbar unter https://www.dge.de/wissenschaft/referenzwerte/vitamin-c/.

[8] Douwes, F. R.: Glutamin. Klinik St. Georg. Bad Aibling. Online verfügbar unter https://www.klinik-st-georg.de/glutamin/.

[9] Vollmer, H. (2004): Kombination entscheidet über Wirkung. Hg. v. Pharmazeutische Zeitung. München. Online verfügbar unter https://www.pharmazeutische-zeitung.de/index.php?id=pharm1_03_2004.

[10] Deutsche Gesellschaft für Ernährung (2020): Empfohlene Tageszufuhr von Zink. Bonn. Online verfügbar unter https://www.dge.de/wissenschaft/referenzwerte/zink/?L=0.

[11] Sauer, B. (2009): IgG Test. Allergologen zweifeln am Sinn. Hg. v. Pharmazeutische Zeitung. Eschborn. Online verfügbar unter https://www.pharmazeutische-zeitung.de/index.php?id=30111.

[12] Bayrischer Rundfunk (2015): Welt in Zahlen-Hormone. München. Online verfügbar unter http://www.daserste.de/information/wissen-kultur/w-wie-wissen/sendung/2010/welt-in-zahlen-hormone-100.html.

[13] Hellhammer, D. (2016): Stress kann man messen. Trier. Online verfügbar unter http://www.stresszentrum-trier.de/fileadmin/img/PDF/20160416_Augsburger_gesundheit_18.04.11.pdf.

[14] Deutsche Gesellschaft für Allergologie und klinische Immunologie (2016): Es bleibt dabei: Keine Empfehlung für IgG(4)-Tests mit Nahrungsmitteln. Berlin. Online verfügbar unter http://www.dgaki.de/es-bleibt-dabei/.

www.ingramcontent.com/pod-product-compliance
Lightning Source LLC
LaVergne TN
LVHW091424190726
843491LV00006B/1598

9783910663008